Gentle Babies

Essential Oils and Natural Remedies for
Pregnancy, Childbirth, Infants and Young Children

REVISED FIFTH EDITION

Debra Raybern

growing
HEALTHY
HOMES

ISBN: 978-0-9816954-8-8
Printed in the United States of America
Fifth printing.

Growing Healthy Homes LLC
P.O. Box 3154
Bartlesville, OK 74006

To obtain additional copies of this book, please visit
www.GrowingHealthyHomes.com.

To Sharon and her future blessings.

To Paul – You are greatly missed.

Dedication

For all the moms and moms-to-be around the globe who wish to choose a more natural approach to motherhood and believe being pregnant is not an illness but rather a joyous time in their lives as they wait for their blessings to arrive.

"Thy wife shall be as a fruitful vine by the sides of thine house; thy children like olive plants round about thy table." - Psalm 128:3

Table of Contents

Acknowledgements

Thank you to the many moms who have used therapeutic-grade essential oils with great success and shared those testimonies and information that have made this book possible.

Thank you to D. Gary Young, N.D., for establishing Young Living Essential Oils, so we may share in the goodness of true essential oils. Without these oils, this book would never have been written.

Thank you specifically to Beverly Boytim, Karen Douglas and Sera Johnson for recording the essential oils and other natural products as they used them to see what worked and what did not.

Thank you to Hasso Wittboldt-Mueller, N.D., whose handout first inspired me to collect more oil information and write this book.

Thank you Laura Hopkins for her editing and design assistance.

Thank you Growing Healthy Homes LLC for publishing this small but awesome book.

Thank you to my daughter, Sharon, who sacrificed the most by allowing her mom the time it took to complete this book.

Thank you to my Lord and Savior Jesus Christ, who put me on a path that included this book.

Debra Raybern

Debra Raybern, N.D., M.H., C.N.C., I.C.A.

Important Information

The pure therapeutic-grade essential oils and natural products referenced in this book are exclusively produced by Young Living Essential Oils (YL). After much careful research and study, it is the opinion of the author and contributors that no other brand of essential oil has the power and purity that is an absolute must for everyone but especially for pregnant and nursing moms and young children.

"Wherefore I put thee in remembrance that thou stir up the gift of God, which is in thee by the putting on of my hands. For God hath not given us the spirit of fear; but of power, and of love and of a sound mind." II Timothy 1:6-7

The Greek word used in this passage for fear is *deilia*, meaning timidity, and its root *deilos* is defined as faithless. This fear is not external but an internal struggle. According to D. Gary Young, founder of YL, "F-E-A-R is a false emotion appearing real." After researching, studying and then selecting the appropriate oil or blend for you or your family, mix with belief and faith that what God made and called "good" is. When used properly and appropriately, like thousands of mothers before you and the over 100 giving their experiences in this book already have, essential oils may prove to provide the benefits you are looking for.

Foreword

In 1991, I became aware of aromatherapy and essential oils when I was searching for complementary and alternative therapies for my daughter. When my little girl was born, she swallowed meconium, the tar-like bowel movement of infants, and it poisoned her system. At seven months old, she had a severe case of pneumonia, and she literally died in my husband's arms as we rushed to the hospital. God miraculously gave her back to us. We lived in critical care unit of the hospital for 10 days.

When she was three, a team of doctors told me she was retarded and nothing could be done for her. I refused to accept their diagnosis and started investigating alternatives in health and nutrition. If someone said they had something to help my daughter, I immediately checked it out. One day, I got a phone call from a friend, Mary, asking if I knew anything about aromatherapy. She told me about the company Young Living, and its founder Gary Young. She suggested I try two essential oils blends, Peace & Calming® and Clarity™. When I found research by Dr. Jean-Claude LaPraz examining the effects of essential oils, I was so impressed I began experimenting with Young Living's essential oils with my daughter. My husband and I were overjoyed as we saw significant, positive changes in her abilities. The changes were so substantial; her teachers and the parents of her friends started asking me what I was doing. It was amazing to watch my daughter's progress. She went from being diagnosed as retarded to graduating from college.

The wisdom I gained over the years enabled me to choose the right information, to grow my mind and to take care of my family and myself. This is why I invest thousands of dollars a year on books, tapes and DVDs that provide knowledge.

Gentle Babies is filled with knowledge of the most important nature; it is about you and how to take care of yourself and your family with essential oils and natural remedies. This wonderful, innovative book by a gifted, generous and intelligent writer will support you and your family with the use of essential oils in your everyday lives. I wholeheartedly recommend it to every family to better their health and as an added resource in their home.

— Marcella Vonn Harting, Ph.D.
Psychoneurology & Integrative Medicine

•••••

The use of essential oils dates back to ancient times; however, there has never been a time when essential oils are more needed in our society than today. The overuse of modern-day 'wonder' drugs has created a potentially hazardous time in our world, more so than the medical science community ever anticipated.

Fortunately, there are answers that provide a way for us to protect ourselves, our family and friends from these potential dangers. The answer is using pure, therapeutic-grade essential oils.

As you can imagine, during our 12 years of using the Young Living products on a daily basis, not only have we gained a better way of life through wellness and longevity, but we also have enjoyed many incredible experiences. As this book has been dedicated to pregnancy, childbirth and infant care, I would like to share some experiences we have had with our grandchildren and the YL products.

We were at our summer cabin and had one of our daughters and her family with us for the weekend. Their youngest son was just a few months old and was suffering from a high fever. I opened my oil bag and proceeded to administer oils on his little body. I used YL's spearmint oil on his back, stomach, forehead and temples and feet several times within an hour. Then, I soaked a wash cloth in cool water with peppermint added and wiped this cloth over him, cooling his body, careful not to make him chill. I also put spearmint in the bath water and let him soak in the tub until the water was cool, then I rubbed R.C.™ on his chest and feet. This broke his fever, and he was back to normal within a couple of hours.

Our youngest daughter used the YL essential oils and supplements throughout her two pregnancies. She used them for nausea and to prevent stretch marks of which she, a petite redhead, has none after two children. She used the supplements to help keep her body functioning properly while giving good nutrition to her baby. She used them at time of labor with great success. She used them at the time of birth, anointing the babies with frankincense right away and using myrrh on the umbilical cords for protection from infections, as well as to help with the healing. She incorporated the oils Debra mentions in this book plus others of her choice as she felt inspired to use them.

We have another grandson who from birth had a runny nose and nothing seemed to help. When he was about three years old, we gave him a drink of NingXia Red®. He liked it and wanted more, and his runny nose stopped and never returned. This was just another confirmation of the power of YL's essential oils and essential-oil-enhanced products.

We became acquainted with Debra many years ago and knew she was someone very special. It has been a delight to see her growth in YL. She has achieved immense success in her search for natural wellness. Her dedication in helping others find natural health and wellness through traditional naturopathic, herbal and essential oils is to be commended.

Well done, Debra. I will consider it a privilege to have your book in my library and will certainly share it with others. I am sure you will see the day when the information contained herein will be mainstay for the masses.

— Shauna Dastrup, friend and associate in the Journey of Health, Wellness and Prosperity

• • • • •

Having had the opportunity to study with Daniel Pénoël, M.D., Jean-Claude LaPraz, M.D., and the physicians at the First Aromatic

Medicine Congress in Grasse, France, I asked these experts about contraindications during pregnancy. I was assured by each of those I interviewed that essential oils are safe for pregnant women and that essential oils could, in fact, offer many benefits.

I often share this information with students in classes so, if a woman realizes she is pregnant, she will not become overly concerned about the oils she might have used before she found out about her pregnancy. In the fourteen years that I have been using and sharing essential oils, I know many, many women who have used essential oils prolifically during pregnancy with excellent results and no observable detrimental effects.

I understand that we may not know everything about essential oils safety, yet, and I encourage women to use oils responsibly and always err on the side of caution. I suggest that women refrain from purposely using substantial amounts of essential oils during pregnancy and use those oils which have withstood the test of time. Additionally, it may be prudent to consider the contraindication lists that have been created in literature available to us and, whenever possible, adhere to these guidelines.

It is time for us to embrace a healing modality which may have profound benefits for women and their families. Debra Raybern has created a book containing a wealth of information about how women everywhere can safely use essential oils to help themselves and their families live longer, healthier and happier lives. On behalf of women everywhere, I thank you, Debra, for writing this book for us.

— Vicki Opfer, C.N.C.

Introduction

"And it came to pass that, when Elisabeth heard the greeting of Mary, the babe leaped in her womb..." Luke 2:41

Pregnancy is one of the most joyful times in a woman's life. At a time when conventional medicine and therapies often are contraindicated, the use of natural protocols and therapeutic-grade essential oils can assist the soon-to-be-mom with a wide variety of health challenges and experiences such as nausea, stress, labor, delivery and afterbirth care for both mom and baby.

Books on the subject of aromatherapy during pregnancy vary widely. One reason for this is the three separate models of aromatherapy: German, British and French. The German model emphasizes inhalation and always extreme dilution. The British model also recommends dilution but concentrates more on the massage benefits. The French model will use both of these and oral ingestion of therapeutic, grade-A essential oils. The work of Daniel Pénoël, M.D., "Natural Home Health Care Using Essential Oils," 1998, showed taking specific essential oils into the body was not only safe but also very effective when other modalities were not.

Essential oil pioneer and globally known expert in the field of growing, harvesting, distilling, blending and usage of essential oils, D. Gary Young has traveled the world learning from each model. As the founder of Young Living Essential Oils (YL), he has combined the best of each model to bring us a unique way of using essential oils plus new, innovative techniques empowering people worldwide to take charge of their health and wellness.

This book combines all modalities, but the safety and effectiveness of these recommendations are found only by using YL's brand of therapeutic-grade essential oils. Because of the purity and quality of these specific oils, the contributors of this book do not endorse any other brand of essential oils.

In the words of Dr. Pénoël, "I'd rather have a single drop of genuine essential oil than a 55 gallon drum of junk product."

All of the recipes and information in this book have been used on thousands of mothers and their babies and children with no ill effects. These have been selected for their safety and effectiveness.

I applaud you for taking the time to learn more about your family's health and how you can use God's original medicine — essential oils — to have vibrant health. Using natural remedies requires more effort than the conventional thinking of "take this pill and call me in the morning." The time you spend will be well worth your health and that of your family.

I hope you will begin to experience the many daily benefits of using essential oils and essential oils products for health, home and body. This is a very self-empowering process; it is a joy to be able to take responsibility for our own health and see the wonderful benefits. Please jot down your notes and findings as you use these products.

It is likely that this book will be a never-ending project as more families benefit from and share their successes. Please share testimonials with us via orders@growinghealthyhomes.com.

Precautions

Young Living Essential Oils (YL), guarantees to provide only 100 percent pure, therapeutic-grade (YLTG™) oils produced from carefully identified plants with natural chemical profiles that match or exceed recognized world standards. In addition, YL has its own more comprehensive, rigorous internal standard, which is an essential prerequisite to gain therapeutic results without producing harmful side effects. This is why I choose YL essential oils.

For Everyone
Avoid citrus oils like lemon, tangerine, grapefruit, lime and bergamot for at least 12 hours to avoid photo-sensitivities on skin areas that are exposed to direct sunlight.

Avoid using skin care products, such as shampoos and lotions, which contain petrochemicals that are counteractive to pure, therapeutic-grade essential oils.

Refer to the Essential Oils Reference guide from www.lifesciencepublishing.com for information on how diet may effect how the oils work.

Pregnancy
Often the following are mentioned in aromatherapy guides as oils to avoid during pregnancy: basil, birch, calamus, cassia, cinnamon bark, hyssop, Idaho tansy, lavandin (a form of lavender often sold in stores as lavender), rosemary, sage, tarragon, and wintergreen. There are a few times throughout this book where a single oil or blend of one of these oils is used. Historically, there have been instances where non-therapeutic-grade essential oils (adulterated, synthetic and of poor quality) have possibly caused a problem during pregnancy. The many moms who have contributed to this book have used all the oils mentioned when appropriate and in the manner listed without problems because they picked the right oil and used it the right way. The difference is quality and common sense.

In her book "*Clinical Aromatherapy: Essential Oils in Practice*," Jane Buckle, Ph.D., R.N., states, "There are no records of abnormal fetuses or aborted fetuses due to the normal use of essential oils, either by inhalation or topical application. There are no records of a few drops of essential oils taken by mouth causing any problem either."

For Babies
For babies (one day to two years old), there are also oils listed to be cautious of or avoid altogether. These include eucalyptus, basil, juniper, peppermint, hyssop and wintergreen. Children are in general more delicate, and some oils such as eucalyptus and peppermint have very strong smells which can, in rare cases, lead to respiratory distress. Be careful when wearing strong smelling oils, diffusing or using around a newborn or young child. Babies also have much thinner, more delicate skin than adults, and tend to be very sensitive to the potency of essential oils. Diluting with a natural lotion is always a good choice. ALWAYS keep essential oils out of reach of children, essential oils are not toys.

For Toddlers and Young Children—2-5 years old
Dilute all essential oils for toddlers and young children. When in doubt, mix a 1:30 blend. This is one part or drop of the essential oil and 30 parts or drops carrier oil, such as YL's V-6™ enhanced vegetable oil complex. Make sure you are selecting the right oil for the issue. A little goes a long way; more is not always better.

Using oils 'neat' or undiluted will create a tendency for the oil to evaporate more quickly. Using a carrier oil or lotion may also create a more sustained effect and reduce possible over-sensitivities especially in this age group.

Sensitivities to YL's essential oils are seen very rarely. Typically, if sensitivities occur, the cause is either that a different brand of chemically adulterated oils were used or because they were used in excess which simply overloaded the system. Food choices, recent vaccinations and family history of health concerns should always be taken into consideration when selecting and using essential oils.

The consensus of opinion on oils safe to use on children include but are not limited to:

- Bergamot (Citrus bergamia)
- Cedarwood (Cedrus atlantica)
- Chamomile, Roman (Chamaemelum nobile)
- Cypress (Cupressus sempervirens)
- Frankincense (Boswellia carteri, sacra)
- Geranium (Pelargonium graveolens)
- Ginger (Zingiber officinale)
- Lavender (Lavandula angustifolia)
- Lemon (Citrus limon)
- Marjoram (Origanum majorana)
- Melaleuca-Tea Tree (Melaleuca alternifolia)
- Orange (Citrus aurantium)
- Rose Otto (Rosa damascena)
- Rosemary (Rosmarinus officinalis)
- Rosewood (Aniba rosaeodora)
- Sandalwood (Santalum album)
- Thyme (Thumus vulgaris CT linalol)
- Ylang Ylang (Cananga odorata)

You are the mom or soon-to-be mom. It is your choice to use or not to use essential oils. If you are more cautious by nature, then by all means dilute the essential oil more, start with smaller amounts or just smell an oil. After all, essential oils are aromatherapy. Even for diffusing in babies room, be sure only a few drops of essential oil is used in a water based diffuser, and run for 10-20 minutes.

As you experience their benefits and confidence grows so will the benefits you receive. As always, before you embark on an essential oil journey, consult with your health care provider, ask questions of other essential oil moms, research, read and, of course, pray.

Just because someone else is doing it one way, doesn't mean that is the correct way for you. The essential oils listed in the Balance Section are ideas based on thousands of moms using essential oils successfully, books on the subject and research. But again, mom and dad — this is your child — not your neighbors, not mine.

When to seek medical attention

While most of the symptoms in this book are everyday ailments mom can confidently handle at home, it is important to know when to seek medical attention.

The following conditions require immediate attention from a midwife or doctor:

• Vaginal bleeding.

• Arterial bleeding, characterized by spurts with each beat of the heart, bright red in color and usually severe and hard to control.

• Lethargy, weakness and difficulty awakening.

• Stiff neck with headache and inability to touch chin to chest.

• Bulging of the baby's fontanel (soft spot on baby's head).

• Broken bones.

• Dehydration, which includes dry lips with dry mouth and no urination for six hours.

• Severe allergic reactions to bee, wasp or other insect stings, producing swelling of the throat and tongue and difficulty breathing.

• Red streaks on the skin emanating from an infection point, possibly indicating blood poisoning.

• Burns that cover more area than the size of the hand, or second or third degree burns that become infected.

• Anything you can't easily fix yourself; seek medical attention.

What are essential oils?

"Every good gift and every perfect gift is from above, and cometh down from the Father of lights, with whom there is no variableness, neither shadow of turning." James 1:17

Essential oils are the aromatic, volatile liquids distilled from plants. The oil can be obtained from the seeds, roots, an entire shrub, flowers, leaves and trees. Each plant may contain hundreds of molecular chemical compounds with names such as terpenes, sesquiterpenes, phenols and aldehydes, to name a few. The Bible contains 188 references to the use of essential oils or the plants from which they are derived.

Essential oils are very complex and currently under much study for their remarkable benefits to our health. For example, clary sage has been found to contain 900 different molecules and lavender over 400.

Like all living things essential oils have a frequency or energy level. Frequency is a measure of the electrical energy that is constant between two points. Bruce Tainio, founder and president of Infinity Resources, Inc., in Cheney, Wash., first developed the technology to measure the frequency of a substance. Plants and their frequencies will vary from plant to plant.

The majority of plant essential oils are obtained by steam distillation to release the plants' precious oil. Only one company — Young Living Essential Oils (YL) — has earned my trust and endorsement. YL's sophisticated and proprietary steam distillation process uses low heat, proper pressure, precise timing and, of course, fresh, properly grown and harvested plants to deliver essential oils with quality and purity unmatched in today's market.

Here is an example of the importance of precise timing during distillation. Cypress has 280 known chemical constituents, and all 280 constituents must be present for cypress to have healing potency. If it is distilled for 20 hours, only 20 of the 280 properties are released. If distilled for 26 hours, none of the properties are released. Most cypress available on the U.S. market is distilled for about three and a half hours. The correct length of time for distilling cypress is 24 hours, releasing all 280 properties.

Also, think about this: it takes 5,000 pounds of rose PETALS to make just one pound of therapeutic-grade rose essential oil. This equates to a truckload of petals. Any rose oil that is inexpensive is basically useless due to synthetic adulteration and will likely pose a health hazard.

YL essential oils go through numerous in-house and independent lab tests and are graded to meet or exceed Association Francaise de Normalisation (AFNOR) standards and International Organization for Standardization (ISO) standards. They are never adulterated, synthetic or chemically enhanced. YL's own internal standard, based on over 30 years of research and study, developing possibly the world's largest essential oil standard library, uniquely enable them to produce only the finest quality product. If they do not make the grade, they are not given the YL label.

Cheap, synthetic, diluted oils are potentially toxic. Therefore, it is very important to use only high-quality essential oils from a trusted source — like right from the farms. YL, the largest producer of therapeutic-grade essential oils in the world, has over 9,000 acres of aromatic farmland where properly grown, harvested, distilled, bottled and blended oils are produced.

The old adage — you get what you pay for — is especially true in the essential oil industry.

How to use essential oils

"All thy garments smell of myrrh, and aloes (sandalwood), and cassia, out of the ivory palaces, whereby they have made thee glad." Psalm 45:8

There are many ways to enjoy essential oils while pregnant, for newborn care and with young children. The Balance Guide of this book lists specific oil ideas and the application methods.

A general guideline when using essential oils is responses should occur relatively quickly. If nothing happens for a while after properly applying an oil, try another oil that works in a similar fashion. While humans are the same species, we still are biologically different and therefore will respond differently to natural products, such as essential oils.

Furthermore, some people are more sensitive than others. Because essential oils are highly concentrated natural plant substances, often it is not the amount of essential oil used at any given application, but the natural frequency of the oil that creates powerful results. This is one reason natural remedies differ vastly from Western medicine because the strength of an essential oil comes through their ability to change the body and the emotions getting to the root of the issue, rather than just an isolated single function or symptom.

Regarding dilution, use a carrier oil such as Young Living Essential Oils' V-6™ enhanced vegetable oil complex, olive oil, almond oil, coconut oil, jojoba oil or other organic plant-based fatty oil. Please note that fatty oils, unlike aromatic oils, can become rancid. Pure aromatic oils stored in a cool, dry place in dark amber or colored glass bottles will not become rancid.

A treadmill will not help someone lose weight if it's not used daily; neither can a person experience the full benefit of essential oils without regular use. The information and ideas contained in this book provide detailed instructions for each chosen application.

CARRIER OILS

Why use a carrier oil? Many people choose to use essential oils "neat," meaning undiluted on themselves and children, but, the real truth is, that just because we CAN does not always mean this is the best method of application. Essential oil use is aromatherapy at its most potent state. Even the mildest of essential oils are very strong and concentrated, so there are times when even one drop is more than what is needed; therefore diluting with a carrier oil becomes the best choice in application. Dilution is not just for topical use but may also be used for inhaling, especially if you are sensitive to smells, have a lifetime exposure to home and environmental toxins or if new to the world of aromatherapy.

There are many carrier oils to select from. Mostly this will be personal preference. When *Gentle Babies* lists the words "carrier oil," feel free to use the one you prefer. As with all carrier oils which come from the fruit or nut of its name, these do not have the long shelf life of essential oils. Storing carrier oils in the refrigerator or a cool cabinet of the home will help them last longer. If ever the carrier oil or blend you have made with a carrier oil smells rancid, do not use it. Be sure to always label the name of the blend you are creating, plus its ingredients and date made. A separate journal or notes in the back of this book are to record your variations on the recipes given. When possible choose organic, lesser refined carrier oils. As with any blending recipe, make small amounts.

Even though you may need to buy a larger bottle of the carrier oils you use, be sure to have a dropper bottle labeled for each when it comes to making a blend as many times the amount needed will be measured in drops, not teaspoons, tablespoons or ounces.

Almond oil, from the almond nut, is nourishing and soothing properties for the skin. Suitable for babies and adults alike, as long as you nor your baby have nut allergies, almond oil is a good choice.

Avocado oil, from the flesh of the avocado (the part we eat), is often combined with one or two other carrier oils. It is very nourishing to the skin and is generally thicker than other carrier oils, which is why it is often combined with olive or almond oil.

Coconut oil, from the flesh of the coconut (the part we eat), can be very nourishing to the skin. If you as the mom can use coconut oil without breakouts or dashing that may occur in some people (it has a tendency to clog pores), then feel free to use some as your carrier oil.

Grape seed oil is a more astringent oil and not generally used alone as the carrier oil on infants and young children, unless this astringent quality is called for.

Jojoba oil is more of a wax than oil, though it is in a liquid state. Great for scalp concerns and softening to the skin, jojoba oil is used in small amounts with other carrier oils.

Olive oil, from the fruit, is a great choice for dry skin that needs rejuvenating and nourishing. The smell may take center stage, so it is often used in conjunction with other carrier oils. Use only organic, first cold press, virgin olive oil.

Rose hip seed oil should only be used in very small amounts in combination with other carrier oils. This is a very regenerative healing oil, useful for scarring and other skin conditions.

Sesame seed oil, from the sesame seeds, has a very powerful odor and best left to small amounts in combinations with other carrier oils or left out completely.

Sunflower seed oil, from the sunflower seed, has minor skin nourishing properties. While suitable in combination with other carrier oils, it may not be your best choice.

V-6™ oil from Young Living contains the following carrier oils for the perfect blend: This is what will be listed in the Balance Guide as the first choice for blending, but, should you or a family member be allergic to one of its components, choose from another carrier oil from this list.

Wheat germ oil is very nourishing to the skin, hair and scalp. Please note: if you have wheat or gluten sensitivities, do not use wheat germ oil.

Carrier oils not suited for infants and young children include castor oil, soap grade coconut oil or cooking oils such as canola oil, corn oil, vegetable oil or sunflower oil.

INHALING

Your oils have just arrived. You're anxious and excited to give them a try. STOP! Even if you are a long time essential oil user, following these first steps with any new oil will make for an even better oil experience.

Open the bottle, and place it at your waist. Let the vapors begin to be released into the air. After 15 seconds, using a swirling motion, raise the bottle up to the chest as you begin to breath deeply. Hold here for one minute.

Lift the bottle to be two to three inches just below your nose, say chin level. Close the left nostril by pressing your finger to the side of the nose and take a slow, deep inhale — no snorting! That may actually cause some oil to go up the nose, and it can burn. It's not hurting you, but it may hurt. Just breathe in and out a few times. Then change and hold the right nostril closed and smell from the left nostril in the same way.

Now, with both nostrils, take several normal breaths.

This process only takes a couple of minutes, but it gets your brain and body accustomed to the oil. Do this with only one or two oils at a time to prevent sensory overload. Now you can add one drop of each of the oils you smelled to a cold air diffuser to run for about 15-20 minutes to let the vapors release into the whole house. Repeat this with no more than two new oils daily. This process does several things. It tells your brain and body — here I come. I'm new and different. But remember me; I'll be using you often. It also begins a slow release of toxins physically and emotionally. It is true; this process can bring up past memories, some pleasant, some not so. If you experience negative emotions, now is a good time to continue using that oil for a few weeks while you address and release these negative emotions.

If you should begin to get a headache or feel short of breath during this process, stop. Go outside and breath in some fresh air while it subsides. Looks like some detoxing may be in order. If you wear contacts and your eyes water, stop the process and do not diffuse right away.

As you become accustomed to essential oils, another inhaling method is to place two to three drops of the oil in the palm of the hand, rub together gently in a clockwise motion, cup hands over the nose and mouth and inhale slowly for six to eight minutes. Up to three oils may be used at a time. Oils travel through the nasal passages into the lungs and according to some research, on to cells in the body and also pass into the brain via the limbic system.

Some people experience physical changes, mental alertness, clarity, relaxation, emotional release and much more just by inhaling the oils. Diluting an essential oil for inhaling is not generally necessary but does not alter the effectiveness of an oil. They also can be smelled straight out of the bottle. Inhale slowly and steadily. Do not snort the oil, as the vapors can irritate the nasal passages and, while no harm is done, this can cause temporary discomfort. If the scent is overpowering, you may dilute with carrier oil or diffuse.

Inhaling is reportedly good for headaches, nervous conditions, anxiety, restlessness, energy, stamina, concentration, cardiovascular challenges and respiratory conditions. In fact, aromatherapy is the science of smell and how it affects the body, mind and spirit.

Again, please note that smelling through inhaling, diffusing and topical application may bring up old memories — some good, some not so good. This is a great time to deal with those negative emotions that may prevent an individual from achieving his or her highest potential by forgetting the past and moving forward.

A Noble Prize for Physiology or Medicine was awarded to Richard Axel, M.D., and Linda Buck, Ph.D., in 2004 for their perceptive discovery of the human genome, specifically the odorants receptors for the sense of smell and the organization of the olfactory system (Nobelprize.org, 2004). The amount of human genome dedicated to smell is many folds larger than any other human genome.

DIFFUSING

A cold-air diffuser is highly recommended to most effectively disperse the oil's hundreds of molecules into the air. A cold air diffuser does no harm to the molecules; while heat may change the chemical structure of the molecules, rendering the therapeutic and healing properties ineffective.

Place four to 10 drops of oil into the diffuser's well, and let it run for about 15 minutes twice per day. The diffuser can be moved from room to room to truly clean the air and make a room smell great. Diffusing may cut the duration of a cold and, in some homes, can actually prevent illness. For example, YL's Thieves® blend was tested at Weber State University (1997) for its potent antimicrobial properties. Thieves® was found to have a 99.96 percent kill rate against airborne bacteria, viruses, mold and fungi.

When using a humidifier, fill the humidifier with water and then place a tissue or cloth sprinkled with a few drops of oil in front of the escaping vapor. Since essential oils can dissolve petrochemicals (plastics), placing the drops of oil directly into the humidifier may cause it to degrade over time.

TOPICAL

The word neat means to apply the oils without diluting. For instance with a bug bite, simply apply one or two drops of bug-bite blend, Purification® blend or KidScents® Bite Buster™ blend oil onto the skin and rub it around. It is recommended to dilute oils for application to small children and babies until skin sensitivity is known. More is not always better with essential oils; they are very powerful by the drop. Only use essential oils in very diluted form in the genital area and on mucus linings as some might sting if not diluted with a carrier oil such as YL's V-6™ enhanced vegetable oil complex or any vegetable oil. This goes for adults as well.

Perform a skin patch test on your forearm to see if you are sensitive to an essential oil. You may wish to dilute more or select a different oil listed. Moms, always use the oil on yourself first before applying to children. If it is hot on your skin, chances are it will be on your children's.

If an essential oil is applied topically and the skin begins to turn red, itchy or hot, add olive oil, V-6™ oil or other carrier oil (page 22) until there is relief. Nothing may be wrong; the oil just brought blood to the skin's surface quickly. This also may occur to those in the habit of using chemical cleansers and soaps, cosmetics, lotions and such with synthetic ingredients, which penetrate the dermal layers of the skin. Applying essential oils to these areas may cause skin irritations and can take these toxins deep into the skin. YL offers a variety of all-natural personal care products for people and pets. If redness occurs, discontinue use, wash the area and apply carrier oil a few times per day until redness subsides. The feet are a great place to start oiling. They almost never develop any redness yet can be quite effective.

Essential oils can be used for all sorts of ear and eye complaints.

For the ears: Apply the suggested oil to the outer back area, under the ear lobe and down the throat to relieve an earache. A cotton ball with a few drops of oil tucked in the ear can also relieve earaches. Oils should not be dropped directly into the ear canal.

For the eyes: Oils should never be used directly in the eye. To support optical wellness, use oil only on the boney area around the eye and across the bridge of the nose. Many people have reported improved eyesight and sty and pinkeye relief by using essential oils at both full strength or diluted. Though it will not cause damage, if oil is accidentally put in the eye, it will sting for a bit and most likely cause the eye to water. For immediate relief, place a drop of V-6™ into the corner of the eye to absorb the essential oil. Never rinse with water as oil and water do not mix, and the oil will spread further.

Vita Flex is a special technique similar to reflexology, using essential oils on various pressure points on the bottom of the feet. Some people are surprised at the results achieved by adding oils to the feet. Dilution, even on children, is generally not necessary on the feet. Consult a reference book for complete instructions.

Bath time can be very relaxing with essential oils. Combine one cup Epsom salts with one cup non-refined salt (optional, but not recommend for those with hypertension) and then add five drops of the oil of choice. Stir to fully spread the oil throughout. Add ½ cup of this mixture to very warm or hot running bath water. Relax, and let the cares of the world melt away. You may replace either or both of the salts with two tablespoons of carrier oil to three drops of essential oil to evenly disperse the oils.

Sitz baths are great for hemorrhoids or stitches after childbirth. Combine three to four drops of essential oils with one tablespoon olive oil and add to warm bath water. Continue to add hot water to keep the bath water warm. Consult your healthcare provider to be sure a bath is allowed.

Hand and foot applications also are beneficial. For nails, combine one ounce V-6™ oil with one drop of essential oil, such as myrrh, lemon oil or frankincense, and one tablespoon whole milk (for the protein). Add this to two cups warm water and let hands or finger tips soak until the water cools. Another application is to bottle the nail oil blend and apply to the nails nightly. For feet, add lavender (lavendula andustafolia) to ¼ cup Epsom salts to a basin of hot water and soak. For any type of foot or nail fungus, add melaleuca alternafolia, Melrose™, Purification® or an anti-fungal blend (see recipe section for options).

Compresses often are used to drive oils deep. Select oils, drop into the hand, mix in a clockwise motion and apply to the area. Then cover the area with a warm wet cloth and top that with a warm dry cloth. Leave it on until it is cool. This is often used for sore achy muscles but may not be warranted during pregnancy or on children under five years of age.

INFANT MASSAGE

One of the many benefits to infant massage includes promoting bonding. Over the years, baby massage also has shown beneficial in assisting overall growth and development, sound sleep, relaxation and reduced fussiness. Additional benefits include relief from the discomforts of gas, colic and digestive complaints. Improvements in respiratory, circulatory and immune system function also have been reported. Gentle massage, using therapeutic-grade essential oils diluted in high-quality carrier oils, is enjoyable for both baby and mom or dad. Parents find the special quality time with baby develops a special bond and using essential oils to support the baby's health give parents confidence in their ability to respond to the child's needs.

Cross-cultural studies show that babies who are held, massaged, carried, rocked and breastfed grow into adults that are less aggressive and violent and more compassionate and cooperative. Recent research shows benefits for premature infants and children with asthma and diabetes. Mothers with postpartum depression have shown improvement after starting infant massage.

Think of the baby massage as a gentle stroking of the body, not the vigorous, deep tissue, Swedish variety. Ideally, both the parent and baby should be in a calm, relaxed state. However, massage also can help calm a baby; a fussy child may respond well to a massage with lavender or Peace & Calming® oil. This may be before bath or bedtime. It is best to wait at least one hour after the baby's feeding.

For specific instructions on massage oils and blends, see the Massage section of the Balance Guide on page 72.

The room should be warm, rather than cool. A temperature of about 78 degrees is good. The baby should lay on his or her back on a padded blanket or towel. The parent can either stand over the baby if using a bed or massage table or sit on the floor with the parent's legs forming a diamond shape where the baby can lie with his head cradled in the adult's feet. Leave the diaper on, but uncover the baby's arms, legs and torso. Be sure to remove all jewelry so as not to scratch the baby.

The parent should place four to five drops of the massage oil or blend in his or her hands and rub together to warm both the hands and the oil. Apply the oil with long gentle strokes on the arms, legs and then torso. Make the strokes gentle but not ticklish. The direction of the massage can be in both directions but end with stokes toward the heart. In the case of digestive concerns (colic, gas, etc), massage in small circles from the right to the left side of the body — the same direction the colon flows. If massaging the scalp, use small circular motion as if shampooing the baby's hair.

During the massage it is fine to softly talk or pray, hum, sing and/ or play soft music. To further bond with the baby, maintain eye contact during the baby massage.

The massage may last 10 to 30 minutes, depending on the mood of the child and the desired results of the massage. Keep a warm towel or blanket nearby to cover the massaged area and keep baby from becoming chilled.

Massage may be done near or around the naval area and spine, but do not focus on these areas. Every parent is capable of giving his or her baby a wonderful massage. A great way to learn more about baby massage is to find a massage therapist skilled in baby or infant massage to teach specific techniques depending on a child's health challenge.

If gas is an issue, hold the legs under the knees, then gently press the knees up toward his or her tummy. This position can help the baby to expel gas.

Hair and scalp massage can be very helpful for healthy hair and scalp. Select the oils from those mentioned in a reference book and combine ½ tablespoon V-6™ oil or wheat germ oil or other carrier oil and five to 10 drops of essential oil. Dip finger tips in the oil and massage into scalp. Cover with warm towel for 20 to 30 minutes, then shampoo as normal. The YL shampoo and conditioner products are loaded with essential oils for specific hair types. These are very concentrated and will not require as much as previously used products, making them very cost effective. Also, adults and children over 12 may use the essential oils neat to clean scalp and hair.

Another massage technique, exclusive to YL, is the Raindrop Technique (RT). A full explanation can be found in the "Essential Oils Desk Reference" (EODR) or "Reference Guide for using Essential Oils." Both are excellent reference books on the use of therapeutic-grade essential oils, with emphasis on the Young Living product line. In a nutshell, RT is a set of specific oils gently applied to the spine and feet. Learn the technique by buying YL's RT kit, which comes with a training DVD and give the whole family the Raindrop experience.

Heavily diluted oils may be used for serious health issues in young children. Contact a massage therapist qualified to perform RT on children. The Center for Aromatherapy Research and Education, raindroptraining.com, has a listing of certified instructors who may be able to refer clients to certified RT therapists.

A modified RT can be useful for infants, but the giver should be proficient with general baby massage with the oils before attempting a RT. Parents should meet with a therapist for individualized instruction. The most important aspect is extreme dilution, avoiding the warm compress and no neck involvement. Most moms find that giving a baby a regular massage and then applying the diluted RT oils to the baby's feet provides the desired results.

HOMEMADE OINTMENTS
Those who do not make their own herbal base can use the Young Living Rose Ointment™, a mildly scented essential oil ointment for topical use that is ideally suited for enhancing with more essential oils to create a personal blend.

Collect the following:
- Two ounce container of Rose Ointment™
- Essential oils based on recipe from Balance Guide — about 10 drops for two ounces of Rose Ointment™. (Do not use more than eight single oils or three blends in these creations unless listed in the recipe. Total oil drops should not be over ten.)
- Small stainless steel sauce pan (one cup is ideal)
- Label for container
- Optional — smaller jars (such as sanitized baby food jars) for lip balms or for sharing. If using smaller jars (one ounce or 1/4

ounce), mix the melted Rose Ointment™ and the essential oils in a glass measuring cup to pour into the smaller containers.

1. Scoop two ounces of Rose Ointment™ into the saucepan.
2. Drop the essential oils from the recipe into the empty Rose Ointment™ container. (Do not wipe the container clean, just use a blunt knife or spatula to empty most of the contents.)
3. Warm the Rose Ointment™ on medium to high heat until melted. Remove from heat and let cool two to five minutes. Move the pan around so to get everything melted on the lowest heat possible.
4. Pour melted Rose Ointment™ back into its container with the added essential oils. The melted Rose Ointment™ automatically will mix with the added essential oils.
5. Let sit uncovered until solid; this should take approximately one hour depending on room temperature. Do not place mixture in the refrigerator or freezer to hasten this process. This will result in a hole in the middle of the jar.
6. Label and use.

Those using Young Living's proprietary Ointment as the base may freely use, share and give away but may not make any for resale.

INTERNAL USAGE

Oral ingestion is safe with nearly every YL essential oil, BUT, BUT, BUT — just because it may be safe to do, it may not be the most effective way to use that oil. If you have a bug bite, are you going to apply the oil topically or take it internally?

When an oil is listed to bring the body back into balance, and ingestion is the application method, put a few drops into an empty capsule, cap and swallow with water. Capsules come in many sizes, with the two most common "0" and "00." These may be purchased at most health food stores or through Young Living. This may be diluted 1:1 or greater with olive oil. It is acceptable to place the oils in a small spoonful of maple syrup, honey or Young Living's Blue Agave or Yacon Syrup or add to almond or rice milk or on a cracker or piece of bread and ingest.

Ingestion may be beneficial for intestinal issues, supportive of the immune system, digestion, endocrine system balancing and a host of other body functions. The FDA has a designation of GRAS — general regarded as safe for those essential oils they regard as safe — for oral consumption. If pregnant or nursing, consult your health care provider before ingesting essential oils.

Oral care should not be neglected. Noel Claffey, M.Dent.Sc., Dean of the Dublin Dental School and Hospital in Ireland, authored a study titled "Essential Oil Mouthwashes: A Key Component In Oral Health Management," which was featured in the Journal of Clinical Periodontology in June 2003. This showed that rinsing with essential oils was better protection against gum disease than flossing. YL carries toothpaste and mouthwash containing the Thieves® blend. To make mouthwash with different essential oils, combine two to three drops of essential oil in one ounce of purified water; then mix, gargle and either spit or swallow. Also, add a drop of Thieves® to the toothbrush for an exhilarating brushing experience, freshening breath for hours.

Retention implants or boluses for vaginal or rectal implanting is largely reserved for more serious health concerns and not recommended while pregnant.

FOOD PREPARATION

Families can have loads of fun preparing food, cooking and making drinks with essential oils. YL's monthly newsletter features several recipes using the YL oils, plus the company offers two cookbooks for healthier essential oil food preparation ideas. Add a drop of cinnamon oil to a batch of oat bran muffins. Put basil and dill in salad dressings and sauces. Blend YL's Yacon Syrup and lemon oil into iced water and stir for delicious lemonade.

With strong oils, such as oregano, even one drop may be too strong. Take a toothpick, insert in the bottle and then stir into the finished sauce, adding more to taste. It is best if the food is not heated in the oven to retain more than just flavor.

HOUSE CLEANING

Cleaning the non-toxic way with essential oils provides much more than a great smell. Most commercial products contain ingredients that can be harmful to people and pets. For a guide to household toxins, refer to the book *Nutrition 101*. The "Labels and Household Toxins" handout is one of many useful charts and articles. The very concentrated Thieves® Household Cleaner is great for walls, floors, kitchens, baths, baby's room and more. Concentrated for cost effectiveness, when tested at Weber State University, the oil Thieves® used in this cleaner had a kill rate of 99.96 percent versus bacteria, fungus, mold and viruses. Lemon oil is another great choice; mix it with a little baking soda for a scouring cleaner.

The Material Safety Data Sheet states — "Thieves® Household Cleaner. Section V, HEATH AND HAZARD DATA, INGESTION: Ingestion of concentrate is not recommended, but no special precautions are needed. If small amounts are consumed, drink water to get rid of the taste."

• • • • •

Some oils may be photosensitizing, meaning they can cause a sunburn if applied in excess and then exposed to the sun. Potentially photosensitizing oils include ginger and citrus oils such as lemon, tangerine, bergamot, and orange.

Before using an oil, always skin test the oil on a small area of the skin first. For babies and children, the feet are a great place to start. Start slowly with diluted oils on other areas, using no more than two or three oils at once.

Research into the effectiveness of essential oils is ever increasing. A simple search on the Internet reveals thousands of scientific, peer reviewed articles validating the effectiveness and safety of using essential oils. Don't take my word for it; I am not responsible for your family's health choices — YOU ARE.

Loss of Pregnancy

If you suspect you are having a miscarriage, please consult your health care provider immediately.

A miscarriage is the loss of a pregnancy during the first 20 weeks. It is usually the body's way of ending a pregnancy that has had a difficult start. The loss of a pregnancy can be very hard to accept. A woman may wonder why it happened or blame herself, but a miscarriage is no one's fault. Essential oils may be useful in the emotional support aspect of losing a child. See the Emotional Support section on page 59 of the Balance Guide.

Preventing some miscarriages may be as simple as additional progesterone. Early in pregnancy, progesterone is made in the ovary called the corpus luteum. After nine to 10 weeks, the placenta should be producing enough progesterone to support the pregnancy. Low levels of progesterone that cause miscarriage usually is thought to be from inadequate production from the corpus luteum. Natural progesterone is considered safe, but studies proving its effectiveness have not been conclusive. If a woman has experienced a previous miscarriage, she should discuss with her health care provider whether progesterone is likely to help with the next pregnancy.

Many bacterial and viral infections can contribute to a miscarriage, including viral infections, such as the cytomegalovirus; bacterial infections, such as chlamydia, mycoplasma and streptococcus; or in rare cases parasitic infection, such as toxoplasmosis. Disease, such as undiagnosed diabetes, also may cause a miscarriage. Chronic illnesses, exposure to environmental toxins (such as certain metals) and stress have also been suspect in some miscarriages. Industry employees working with chemicals such as dyes, metals or solvents are at greater risk. Maternal stresses and heavy use of tobacco, caffeine, alcohol and drugs also are potential factors.

Mothers would do well to eat a nutritious diet well before conception and throughout pregnancy. See the Nutrition Guide on page 88. Prior to conception rid the home of harmful chemical toxins (household cleaners, air fresheners, detergents, bath and body care products, etc.). Using essential oils and essential-oil-based products from Young Living Essential Oils is one way to be confident the cleaning products used in the home are toxic free and safe for all.

Balance Guide

The following wellness concerns listed include several possible balancing ideas for pregnant or nursing women and babies or children. Nearly all the entries below are an essential oil or a product enhanced with essential oils. The topics included in this guide may be common during a normal pregnancy and childbirth. Certain more serious concerns are not included, as they always require professional medical care and intervention.

Before you begin, remember that you are responsible for your family's health. This guide includes holistic alternative ideas, not medical treatment. Most of the concerns are specific for the baby or child and the mom. In the case when the mom or her little one could have the same condition, such as coughs, and congestion, there may be a "For baby" (ages one day to two years old), "For child" (two years to five years) and "For mom" alternative. Typically children up to age five will respond very well with the information for babies, but a separate listing "For Child" includes applications that children over two years old may respond to quicker. As children grow, it may be effective to dilute oils less and apply them more often until the concern is balanced.

***Concerning babies and infants, ages one day to two years: remember that your baby is tiny, fresh into this world, delicate, weighs far less than you and is still growing and forming in many ways. Herbs and essential oils are potent and powerful substances God gave us for the betterment of our health and for protection of the germs and health concerns we might experience. They are not be used in the same way adults do; please keep this in mind. Please read ALL of this book, not just jump into the Balance

Guide. This will better equip you to use essential oils with your family, safely and effectively. A great way to use the oils in infants and young children is simply to rub the oils in your hands with a bit of carrier oil then hold over the child's back, chest or feet for a minute or so. Then hold the child's foot for a minute touching the oils to the foot. The oil vapors and frequency are very potent — a little goes a long way in most cases.

Those who choose to vaccinate or use antibiotics with infants and young child/children should consider taking a slower approach to essential oil usage until the child/children are a few days away from the vaccine or finished with antibiotic treatment. This is because pharmaceuticals may alter the body's immune system, which the oils will strive to rebalance. This also may initiate a response considered by those without an understanding of the chemistry of Young Living Essential Oils to be an adverse reaction to the oils. On the contrary, the oils are performing their natural function intended by God to help the body find a healthy balance. Nutritional and supplemental support of the elimination system may be a wise choice to further aid the rebalancing.

Mothers may choose one or use multiple suggestions, as balancing has been reported with each. If a mother selects more than one essential oil, she should apply the first as directed, then wait 10 minutes. If the desired results are not achieved, then apply the second suggestion. Mothers will no doubt have favorites and should highlight them for future reference.

Many supplements contain warnings against their use when pregnant or nursing. This is mainly because little to no testing is conducted on pregnant or nursing women. Before taking any supplement or using essential oils, please consult with your midwife, doula or other healthcare provider looking after you while pregnant.

NOTE ON STUDIES: Many cautions or lists to avoid are based on research of a specific, often synthetic compound — NOT the whole, pure, therapeutic essential oils. YL essential oils are NOT toxic. Any reaction you get may simply be the body manifesting an underlying issue you need to take care of.

STOP — before reading further — here are a few rules to follow:
1. If you think medical attention is needed, then get it.
2. Posting a photo on social media and asking for diagnosis or asking for recommendations is NOT equal to medical attention.
3. STUDY the reference books and create your own family medicine chest of ready to use, diluted, labeled essential oils.
4. Know the single oils used in the blends you choose.
5. Choose alternatives to cautionary essential oils, if you are in fear.
6. Use the smallest amount and repeat if needed.
7. Apply properly — this means diluted until you know a stronger application is appropriate for you or baby.
8. Use common sense. If it does not feel right to you, then do not do it.

PREGNANCY—General Information
This is a most amazing time in a woman's life, and no doubt many will share their experiences and advise with you. Moms — this is your baby; YOU must weigh all the advise and take only what you and your health care provider deem appropriate. Books abound sharing — use this, use that — including this one based on both research and the experience of hundreds of moms. There may be someone who reacts poorly, but as stated on page 15, there has yet to be any record or an aborted or damaged fetus from the proper use of essential oils. Reactions are the oil bringing up an underlying problem that needs to be addressed.

From the available books, there are essential oils suggested to either avoid or use with caution. Why? Because the research on these so called oils was based on synthetic chemical compounds, NOT the complete oil God created. BUT have been used by thousands of moms with great success. I pray you have a healthy, happy pregnancy.

ACID REFLUX (also see INDIGESTION and COLIC for infants)

For Mom:

AlkaLime®—Mix one tsp in water in the morning and evening on an empty stomach. Also may be taken after a meal if indigestion causes discomfort.

Peppermint—One drop on tongue or in a glass of water.

Peppermint has been reported by some nursing moms to cause a reduction in milk supply. Some aromatherapy texts suggest avoiding during pregnancy and while nursing.

AFTER BIRTH, Care for and Anointing Baby (also see LABOR AND DELIVERY and TRAUMA)

Mix any oil of choice below with 30 drops to one ounce natural lotion or carrier oil and apply 1-3 drops of the mixture as follows:

Frankincense—Apply a few drops diluted to the head as an anointing oil.

Trauma Life™—Apply a few drops diluted on the crown of the head and the feet soon after birth.

Valor®—Apply to feet. Wait five or 10 minutes before using another oil.

Brain Power™, Joy™ or Peace & Calming®—Apply diluted to feet.

Lavender—Apply diluted to feet for relaxation when needed.

Myrrh—Apply a few drops diluted to the body as an anointing oil with a lotion or carrier oil.

Gentle Baby™—Place two to four drops diluted on abdominal area.

AFTER BIRTH CARE FOR MOM

If mom has previously used essential oils, dilution may not be needed.

ClaraDerm™ Spray—Apply as needed on vaginal area.

Gentle Baby™—Place two to four drops on abdominal area.

Frankincense—Apply to the head as an anointing oil.

Trauma Life™—Apply on the crown of the head and the feet right after birth. Smell also.

Valor®—Apply to feet. Wait five or 10 minutes before using another oil.
Brain Power™, Joy™ or Peace & Calming®—Apply to feet.
Lavender—Apply diluted to feet for relaxation when needed.

ALLERGIES
For pregnant mom:
Lavender, R.C.™ and eucalyptus radiata—Diffuse 20 to 30 minutes twice per day or as needed.
Eucalyptus radiata—Put one drop or less on the pinky finger and swab the inside of the nose but not deeply.

For mom:
Lavender—Five drops in a capsule and ingest between meals.
Eucalyptus radiata—Put one drop or less on the pinky finger and swab the inside of the nose but not deeply.

For children over two-years-old:
Eucalyptus radiata—Put one drop or less on the pinky finger and swab the inside of the nose but not deeply. Diffuse.
Lavender—Ingest one drop in a teaspoon of honey or YL's Yacon Syrup once or twice per day.

Lavender has been working wonderfully for my allergies. I almost can't believe the difference! ~ April

AUTISM
Many children diagnosed with autism and related disorder symptoms improve with diet change and the use of certain essential oils. Reducing high glycemic, non-nutritive foods with wholesome choices also is quite beneficial. The book *Nutrition 101: Choose Life!* guides families to better, more wholesome eating habits that will benefit all family members. See page 116 for ordering information.

Children two years and older:
KidScents® MightyZymes—Use as directed on bottle.
KidScents® MightyVites—Use as directed on bottle.

NingXia Red®—Drink one half to one ounce per day. Dilute in glass of water, if preferred. This is an excellent source of vitamins and minerals, anti-oxidants and glutathione, which autistic children are often deficient in.

Brain Power™, frankincense, Clarity™, Peace & Calming®, Idaho balsam fir, Valor®, cedarwood and sandalwood—Diffuse any or all. May also have the child apply the oil to the scalp and wear as perfume.

> "My son Noah, a five-year-old diagnosed with autism, could not converse with us; he just repeated phrases he'd heard. In May, we made the commitment to give him three MightyZymes each day, every day. By the end of June, he burst out of his shell. He began talking in a conversational method and asking and answering questions. He wanted us with him, to play with him, to watch movies with him and read to him. I believe that through YL's MightyZymes and essential oils, our Heavenly Father has released our child from many of the daily struggles of autism."
> ~ Evon (Read the complete testimony on page 110.)

BABY ACNE

This may occur on the cheeks and sometimes on the forehead, chin and back. Milia are tiny bumps that appear on the face at birth and disappear within a few weeks, and they're unrelated to acne. If the irritation is more rashy or scaly than pimply or it appears elsewhere on the body, the baby may have another condition, such as cradle cap or eczema which would require diagnoses.

Lavender and Melrose™—One drop of each dilute 1:30 or less and apply to affected areas of skin, and be careful to avoid eyes and mouth.

BACK PAIN—For mom (also see MUSCULAR PAIN)
PanAway® or Deep Relief roll-on—Apply directly on area of discomfort.
Valor®—Apply neat or diluted 1:1 on the area.
Aroma Siez™—Apply directly on the area.

BATHING BABY
Use only a mild bath gel or soap on a new baby.
KidScents® Bath Gel—Follow instructions on the bottle.

BED WETTING—Children
Melrose™—Apply diluted or neat over the bladder.
Peace & Calming® and Valor®—Apply to bottom of feet at bedtime.
Remove all carbonated beverages completely as these are acid forming and may irritate the kidneys and bladder, exacerbating this condition. Stop all fluids two hours before bedtime.

"My daughter started taking one Omega Blue™ (now known as OmegaGize³™) capsule each day to help her unexplained bed wetting, a problem she'd dealt with since she was a toddler. Beginning the day she started taking Omega Blue™ (now known as OmegaGize³™), she has never wet the bed again; it was that effective" ~ Sera

BLADDER VOIDING AFTER BIRTH
Occurring during late pregnancy and sometimes after giving birth or a C-section, there may be a time when the woman is unable to void her urine.
Add one drop of **peppermint** to the toilet bowl and have the woman sit on it immediately. Another option is to rub one drop **eucalyptus** over the bladder. Many midwives report success using one or the other of these oils.

BLEEDING, spotting, for mom:
If bleeding vaginally, consult with a midwife or doctor immediately.
Shock Tea—For this home remedy, use one cup warm water, three tablespoons apple cider vinegar and one teaspoon cayenne pepper and three tablespoons honey (optional). Stir all together and drink with a straw.
Helichrysum—Put one drop under the tongue every 10 minutes as you seek medical attention.

Trauma Life™—Apply externally to the wrists and inhale to reduce the stress of the issue while seeking medical attention.

BLEEDING, minor on skin, for baby or children:
Tsuga—Apply externally on location.
Geranium—Apply one to two drops directly for any bleeding around umbilical cord/belly button. This may be diluted. Consult healthcare provider.
Rose Ointment™—Apply topically to the area.
Helichrysum—Apply one to two drops **helichrysum** to the skin where the bleeding is happening. Apply slight pressure and repeat if needed. Consult healthcare provider.
NOTE: With bleeding on the skin, wash with clean, cool water and then cover with a damp gauze or cloth and apply pressure. Apply tsuga or helichrysum oil to the area and re-cover. Check in five to 10 minutes. If stitches are required, go to the nearest medical facility. In many cases of minor bleeding, the **tsuga** oil and then a small amount of **Rose Ointment™** is all that is required. Clean area to avoid infection.

BLEEDING, minor on skin, for mom:
Tsuga—Apply externally on location.
Rose Ointment™—Apply topically to the area.
Helichrysum—Apply one to two drops **helichrysum** to the skin where the bleeding is happening. Apply slight pressure and repeat if needed. Consult healthcare provider.
NOTE: With bleeding on the skin, wash with clean, cool water and then cover with a damp gauze or cloth and apply pressure. Apply tsuga or helichrysum oil to the area and recover. Check in five to 10 minutes. If stitches are required, go to the nearest medical facility. In almost all cases of minor bleeding, the **tsuga** oil and then a small amount of **Rose Ointment™** is all that is required.

BLOOD PRESSURE/HYPERTENSION
Preeclampsia, also known as pregnancy-induced hypertension (PIH), is a form of high blood pressure occurring only during pregnancy, and all treatment should be supervised by your health

care provider. If they approve, consider:

Aroma Life™—Apply one or two drops on the heart area and inner wrist to normalize. Also inhale.

Ylang ylang—Apply one or two drops on the heart area and inner wrist to normalize. Also inhale.

NingXia Red®—One to two ounces a day to normalize.

Lavender—Inhale every five minutes until normalized.

BLOOD SUGAR (see GESTATIONAL DIABETES)

BOILS

Melrose™—one drop applied directly on the boil once or twice daily. May be diluted 1:1 with carrier oil for younger children and babies.

Thieves® or DiGize™—May be diluted 1:30 with carrier oil for younger children. **Thieves®** and **DiGize™** contain some ingredients listed as cautionary in some texts. **Thieves®** ingredients—clove, lemon, cinnamon bark, eucalyptus radiate and rosemary. **DiGize™** ingredients—tarragon, ginger, peppermint, juniper, fennel, anise, patchouli and lemongrass.

BONDING WITH BABY

Gentle Baby™—Apply one or two drops on the pregnant belly. May be used neat or diluted.

"I used Joy™ to help relieve stress and promote additional bonding because my daughter was premature and spent a week in the neonatal intensive care unit. As a toddler, anytime she is fussy or agitated, I have her inhale Joy™, apply it to her like perfume and say 'the joy of the Lord is our strength.'" ~ Laura

BREAST INFECTION/MASTITIS/MILK FEVER

This may occur if breasts are not emptied completely, when milk ducts get clogged or if breast feeding is abruptly stopped.

Geranium (one drop), lavender (one drop) and Melrose™ (two drops)—Combine oils in 1.5 pints cold water, dip washcloth into mix, squeeze excess water out and apply on breast as a cold compress. Repeat as frequently as each hour during the day.

If fever is associated:

Eucalyptus globulus—Add five drops to ½ teaspoon sea salt to a basin of warm water and soak feet. Repeat as frequently as each hour during the day.

Melrose™—Apply a warm compress to a clogged milk duct. Do this after nursing and wash breasts just prior to the next nursing time.

BREECH BABIES

When the baby has not turned to be vertex (head down) for labor and delivery but is presenting bottom first, the position is termed breech.

Peppermint—Apply to the abdomen. (See midwife testimony on page 100). Use only under supervision of midwife or doula to be sure baby turns in the proper direction.

Myrrh—Apply several drops to the belly and rub them into the skin. Repeating the application may be needed. Use only under supervision of midwife or doula to be sure baby turns in the proper direction.

CESAREAN/C-SECTION

This is a surgical procedure where an incision through the abdomen and uterus is used to extract the baby.

Rose—One drop on closed, healing incision may assist in releasing emotional trauma and is rejuvenating to the skin/tissue.

Helichrysum—One drop on location may help heal tissue trauma and stop minor bleeding.

Lavender—Liberally apply on location may prevent scaring and promote skin healing.

Believe™—One drop diluted on the area for wound healing.

Trauma Life™—Smell to ease emotional trauma.

CHICKEN POX

Chicken pox, or Herpes zoster, is related to the Herpes simplex virus and is highly contagious.

LavaDerm™ Spray—Spray on rash to relieve itching.
Australian Blue™, Roman chamomile, lavender, Melrose™, Thieves® or ravintsara—Apply one drop of selected oil diluted to the bottom of the feet three times daily at onset.
NingXia Red®—Drink one ounce daily.
Raindrop Technique—Refer to the Essential Oils Desk Reference for instructions on this technique, which is very useful for all types of viral conditions including chicken pox, shingles and measles. Consult with an experienced Raindrop therapist for guidelines on this technique with children under age five.

CIRCULATION
For mom:
Aroma Life™, cypress, helichrysum and tangerine oil—Combine a couple of drops of each with several drops of a carrier oil and massage legs daily, or add oils to carrier oil or Epsom salts for a foot soak.
NingXia Red®—Drink one ounce twice a day.
Ortho Ease® Massage Oil—Apply to legs.
Omega Blue™ or OmegaGize³™—Take one to four capsules daily as directed on bottle.

CIRCUMCISION
Rose Ointment™—Apply topically with each diaper change to prevent healing area from sticking to diaper.
Animal Scents™ Ointment—Apply topically, as directed above. Despite the name, **Animal Scents™ Ointment** works well for humans too.

COLD SORE, Moms
Cold Sore Ointment—Use the ingredients below and follow the instructions on page 32 to create this ointment. Apply to the cold sore multiple times a day.
   Lavender (two drops)
   Melissa (two drops)
   Melrose™ (two drops)

Sandalwood (two drops)
Ravintsara (one drop)
Thyme (one drop)

COLIC
This is when an infant has episodes of crying and irritability with what appears to be abdominal pain. Nursing mothers should examine their diet for offending foods and avoid caffeine, foods with high fat content and spicy foods that may be too harsh for the baby.

Roman chamomile—Place one drop in bowl of warm water and soak a washcloth, wring and use as a compress on baby's belly.

Dill, copaiba or frankincense—Place one drop in one tablespoon of either V-6™ oil or carrier oil and rub on the middle of the baby's back in circular, clockwise motions.

DiGize™—Dilute one drop in one teaspoon olive oil rubbed on the baby's abdomen or feet. Contains **fennel**—Avoid if family history of epilepsy or seizures exists.

Peppermint—Dilute one drop in one teaspoon olive oil rubbed on the baby's abdomen or feet. **Peppermint** contains menthol, which has been reported to cause bronchial spasms in rare cases. Dilute further, keep away from babies nose and mouth; or select a different oil if concerned, and if the use of **peppermint** is new to your family.

CONGESTION (also see COUGHING and RESPIRATORY INFECTION)
For babies and children:
Lemon, melaleuca alternafolia, pine, myrtle or cedarwood— Two drops each in one ounce carrier oil applied to upper back and back of neck.

Thieves®—Dilute 1:30 and apply to bottom of feet. Diffuse 1:1 with **lemon** oil for 10-20 minutes.

For older children:
Same as above or **eucalyptus radiata, lemon, R.C.™** or **Purification®**—Diffuse one or all to decongest.

"Not long after my son was born, my family dealt with a nasty upper respiratory virus with major congestion and croupy coughing. Of course, we all increased our NingXia Red® doses up to three to six ounces a day. My daughters, husband and I all took three to five Inner Defense™ capsules a day, and I diffused and applied lots of R.C.™ to our chests, necks and feet helping us get rid of it in about half the time it would have normally taken. However, my five-week-old came down with a low fever and had some congestion which I knew was pretty serious for a newborn. I rubbed R.C.™, diluted 1:1 with V-6™ oil, all over his chest and bottoms of his feet every two hours or so and applied lavender to the bridge of his nose for a blocked tear duct. As I was praying over him, I felt led to apply Frankincense all over his body, around the outside of his eyes and over his sinuses. I also diluted some Thieves® 1:1 and rubbed it on the bottom of his feet. The next day, his fever was gone, the congestion was cleared, and even the blocked tear duct was open and the infection in his eye was totally cleared up!"
~ Sera

CONTRACTIONS (see LABOR)

CONSTIPATION
For babies:
DiGize™, ginger, lavender—Apply diluted 1:30 or less to lower abdomen and bottom of the feet. **DiGize™** contains **fennel**—Avoid if family history of epilepsy or seizures exists

For children:
KidScents® MightyVites and KidScents® MightyZymes—For children who are eating solids, use as directed on bottle.
Peppermint—Dilute one or two drops and apply to the bottom of the feet and rub in circular, clockwise motions.
DiGize™—Apply diluted 1:30 or less to lower abdomen and bottom of the feet. Contains **fennel**—Avoid if family history of epilepsy or seizures exists.

Ginger—Apply neat to bottom of the feet in the center and heel area.

For mom:
Life 5™ Probiotic—This probiotic supplement may assist in proper bowel function. Use as directed on bottle.
ComforTone®—If tendency toward constipation exists, **ComforTone®** capsules before breakfast and bedtime may provide relief. Start with one capsule and increase daily as needed. Follow appropriate nutrition to prevent constipation. (See Nutrition Guide on page 88.) Drink eight or more eight-ounce glasses of distilled water throughout the day for best results. Do not begin taking **ComforTone®** in the last trimester unless instructed by your health care provider.
ICP™—Mix two teaspoons with at least eight ounces of fresh juice or water and drink daily. This contains advanced fibers that scour the colon; increased fiber leads to better bowel formation and movement. Do not take more than one teaspoon per day after third month.
Essentialzyme™—One to three capsules before meals to improve digestion.
Balance Complete™—Add two scoops to eight to 10 ounces of cold water with breakfast and/or lunch. Not to be used as a meal replacement.
NingXia Red®—One to three ounces daily.

COUGHING (also see CONGESTION, RESPIRATORY INFECTION and WHOOPING COUGH)
For babies and children:
Lemon and Purification®—Diffuse several drops of either or both about 15 to 20 minutes in the bedroom before bedtime.
Peace & Calming®, copaiba or myrtle—Place a few drops diluted 1:5 or more on the chest mixed with a few drops of carrier oil. Cover with a shirt or swaddle to avoid strong smell.

For mom:
Lemon oil—Ingest one or two drops in a teaspoon of Grade B Maple Syrup or YL's Yacon Syrup.

Thieves®—Place one to two drops on the bottom of the feet.
Inner Defense™—May use as directed on the bottle.

> "When Joshua was 10 months old, he got a severe upper respiratory virus. I did not have any Young Living essential oils at the time, so that morning I tried the onion and garlic poultice. After the first application, the congestion started breaking up, and he was having productive coughs. Then, a few hours later, I did it again. By that night, his lungs were totally clear, and he slept great!" ~ Sera

CRADLE CAP
The medical term is seborrheic dermatitis, and it describes the inflammation in the upper layers of the skin, causing scales on the scalp, face and occasionally other areas. This condition may be due to low intake of biotin in the mothers diet. Refer to page 115 and *Nutrition 101: Choose Life!* for information of obtaining biotin from food.
Lavender—Dilute or use neat on affected area.
Melrose™—Dilute or use neat on affected area.
Rose Ointment™—Apply to the scalp. It also may be combined with a drop of either, or both, of the oils listed above.

CRYING BABY
Peace & Calming®—Apply diluted or neat to the feet and back of neck. Also have the baby smell the oil from mom or dad's hands waved overhead but not right next to babies nose. Parents and caregivers can also wear on themselves and hold baby and diffuse in the area.
Lavender or Joy™—Have the baby smell the oil from an adult's hands waved overhead but not right next to babies nose. Parents and caregivers can also wear on themselves and hold baby.

"When my newborn is crying and I know he is not hungry, wet, or sleepy, I hold different oils up to his nose for him to smell. Most of the time, he stops crying as he is experiencing this new smell and even settles down as if he forgot why he was crying. By experimenting like this, I have found that one of his favorites is lavender. It really helps to calm him." ~ Sera

DETOXIFYING

Pregnancy and when nursing is not the time to embark on an aggressive cleanse. Once a baby is weaned or at least only nursing a few times per day is generally the time when a mother can begin cleansing. Until then, you may drink one to two servings of **Balance Complete**™ daily (as a snack, not meal replacement), drink Green Smoothies (see page 91 for the recipe) and drink **NingXia Red**® to maintain a mild nourishing cleanse. Also refer to the section on Nutrition Guide on page 88.

DIAPER PAILS (see House Cleaning on page 35)
Thieves® **Household Cleaner**™ may help keep the diaper pail sanitized and smelling fresh for moms using cloth diapers. In one pint of cool water add one capful of **Thieves**® **Household Cleaner**™. Pour into the bottom of the clean diaper pail.

DIAPER RASH
Avoid commercial products that contain irritants such as talc and mineral oil.
Gentle Baby™—Dilute 1:30 with YL V-6™ or almond oil and apply on location.
KidScents® **Tender Tush ointment**—Apply topically.
Animal Scents™ **Ointment**—Apply topically.
Rose Ointment™—Apply topically.
Diaper ointment recipe—Use the ingredients below and follow the instructions on page 32 to create this ointment. Apply multiple times a day.
   Gentle Baby™ (four drops)
   Lavender (two drops)
   German Chamomile (two drops)

Cypress (one drop)
Melrose™ (one drop)
Baby powder alternative—Mix two tablespoons of cornstarch with five drops of either **lavender, rose** or **Gentle Baby™** essential oil. Sift together several times until well blended. Store in a tightly sealed container.
Baby oil alternative—Mix two tablespoons of carrier oil with five drops **lavender** or **Gentle Baby™**. Store in a tightly sealed container.
Homemade baby wipes—Take a roll of natural paper towels, which typically are brown in color and made from recycled paper and contain no chemicals, just 100 percent cotton/natural fibers. Cut the roll in half using a serrated knife. Obtain a clean round container with a tight fitting lid that will hold the half roll. Flatten the roll and then remove the inner cardboard core. Place the half roll in the container. In a separate bowl, add:

2 cups distilled or boiled bottled water that has cooled to room temperature
2 Tbls. **Young Living Lavender Shampoo** or **KidScents® Shampoo**
2 Tbls. V-6™ mixing oil blend
5 drops of any Young Living Essential Oil of choice, such as **lavender, Gentle Baby™, sandalwood,** or **frankincense.**
(Adding essential oils is optional because the Young Living shampoos contain therapeutic-grade essential oils.)
Whisk the mixture together well and pour over the flattened roll in the container. Cover, and let sit overnight to absorb all the liquid. When ready to use, open container and pull a wipe from the center, tear off and use. Close lid securely between uses to avoid drying out. If wipes become dry, add a few tablespoons of sterile water to re-hydrate.

"My three month old had a severe diaper rash. I tried all the normal ointments and was getting no where. One day I put some Burt's Bees on him, and he started screaming. I put him in the bathtub and washed him off and decided to apply some KidScents® Tender Tush. He started laughing at me as I applied it! The rash was gone the next day!" ~ Beverly

DIARRHEA
Babies and children:
Copaiba—Apply one to two drops diluted 1:5 or more over abdomen.

Moms:
DiGize™ or copaiba—Apply one to two drops over abdomen. In addition, adults may put two drops **DiGize™** in water to sip on.
Lavender—Apply one drop of each over abdomen to calm stress induced by diarrhea.
Peppermint—One drop orally. Peppermint may reduce milk supply if nursing.
Ledum—Apply one to two drops over abdomen and take one drop orally.
ICP™—Place a few teaspoons in water to absorb excess water in the colon.
Inner Defense™—Take one capsule per day if a stomach bug is suspect.
Life 5™—Take one or two capsules daily to establish the good gut flora in the system.
Geranium, cypress, sandalwood and Roman chamomile—Apply one to two drops applied over abdomen.

DIETARY REGIMEN DURING PREGNANCY (see NUTRITION GUIDE on page 88)
Follow advise from your healthcare provider and include these as approved.
NingXia Red®—Two to three ounces daily.
Core Supplements™—Take daily as directed.
OmegaGize³™—Take one to four capsules daily as directed on bottle.
Pure water—Ingest half body weight in ounces, plus an additional 20 ounces to avoid swelling in hands, legs and feet. This also helps prevent nausea.
Pure Protein Complete™—Take as directed for extra protein needs, especially for breakfast. Eat lots of fresh vegetables and fruit.

DILATION, if delayed and the health adviser or midwife suggests encouraging dilation

Clary Sage—Massage around the ankle bone or ingest one drop every 15 minutes until dilation begins. Other moms have taken six drops and then take a wait-and-see attitude and reassess after four or five hours. Monitor over the next couple hours. Then repeat if necessary. Do not try to force the delivery.

EAR INFECTIONS
For children:

Lavender, cedarwood or Melrose™—Dilute 1:10 and apply one or two drops all around on the outer ear, down the neck and on the feet several times daily. May place a drop on a cotton ball and place on surface of the ear. These oils may also be applied to the feet.

FOR EXTREME CASES ONLY**—As mentioned previously on page 28, it is not recommended to place essential oils directly into the ear canal. There is an exception, but only under the following conditions: restricted the use of a pacifier; eliminated all milk consumption, including raw cow or goat; making sure the bowels are working properly, meaning two to three times daily; and the above mentioned oils on the outer ear fail to relieve the pain and discomfort. Use the following recipe, making no substitutions including size of dropper bottle or exceptions for safety and effectiveness. Mix the following in an ¼ ounce or less sized dropper bottle:

V-6™ or first cold press olive oil (20 drops)
Lavender (one drop)
Melrose™ (one drop)

Use one drop of this mix in each ear one time per day. It is rarely needed beyond one day.

"My six month old got a really bad ear infection. We took him to the doctor, and, after he went through three rounds of antibiotics, the pediatrician finally suggested an antibiotic injection. I drew the line there, and she said then we would have to go to an Ear, Nose and Throat specialist and get tubes put in his ears. The ENT could not see us for two weeks, so we called a naturopath we had recently meet and asked her what we could do. By now, this infection had been going on for a couple of months and was only getting worse. She told us to remove dairy from his diet, rub ledum below his ear and down his neck, rub Thieves® on his feet and apply colloidal silver in his ear. When we went to the ENT two weeks later, he looked in his ears and said there was no sign of infection. He asked what we had done, and, of course, in his mind, none of it made any difference. I knew that the oils were what killed this infection." ~ Beverly

"My six-month-old was cranky and pulling on her ears so I used the Melrose™ blend in her ear several times a day. I would also applied ledum in a downward motion from her ear to her chin line. She was having a hard time sleeping and was congested as well, so I had her at an incline. After putting the oil in her ears with a teeny bit of cotton ball, she slept for hours and was not cranky. I have now learned if I don't eat much dairy while nursing we can avoid any congestion and ear problems with her. ~ Jeanette

"Our friends were planning to fly again with their two-year-old daughter and did not want to relive a previous flight when she was very agitated and disruptive. They used Peace & Calming® prior to the flight, and the child slept through the night for the first time in weeks. During the flight, the child was calm and the Melrose™ helped alleviate any pressure she and her mom experienced during takeoff and landing." ~ Laura

ECZEMA/DERMATITIS

This is a general term encompassing various inflamed skin conditions. Although it may look different from person to person, it is most often characterized by dry, red, extremely itchy patches on the skin. In infants, eczema typically occurs on the forehead, cheeks, forearms, legs, scalp and neck. In children and adults, it typically occurs on the face, neck, and the insides of the elbows, knees and ankles.

Babies and children:
Lavender and Melrose™—Place two drops in the palm, stir in several drops carrier oil, mix and apply on the affected area.
KidScents® Tender Tush—Apply like lotion over the area.

Mom:
Lavender and Melrose™—Place two drops in the palm, stir to mix and apply neat on the affected area.
KidScents® Tender Tush—Apply like lotion over the area.
Detoxzyme® or Allerzyme™—Use as directed on bottle.
Lemon oil—Apply neat on the affected area.
Lavender and Rose Ointment™—Apply a few drops **lavender** and then top with **Rose Ointment™**.
Lavender Hand & Body Lotion—Slather on the skin.
Irritated skin ointment—Use the ingredients below and follow the instructions on page 32 to create this ointment. Apply as needed.
   Lavender (two drops)
   German Chamomile (one drop)
   Cistus (one drop)
   Palmarosa (three drops)
   Geranium (two drops)
   Helichrysum (one drop)

EDEMA/WATER RETENTION
This includes swelling usually in the legs, feet and ankles.
Cypress and tangerine oil—Add one drop of each to drinking water. Repeat several times a day.
NingXia Red®—Drink one to two additional ounces daily.
Water Retention Massage Oil Blend:
   Tangerine oil (two drops)
   Lemon oil (one drop)
   Cypress (four drops)
   Lavender (four drops)
   Geranium (three drops)

Mix oils into two and ½ tablespoon almond oil, ½ tablespoon jojoba oil and one Evening Primrose carrier oil capsule (approximately 10 drops). This may be used all throughout pregnancy. Relax on the sofa with legs raised on pillows. Apply the oils to feet, ankles and legs, massaging toward the heart to help circulation. You may substitute carrier oil of your choice for the three mentioned.

EMOTIONAL SUPPORT (also see FEAR, PANIC, POSTPARTUM DEPRESSION, SELF-LOVE, SELF-ESTEEM and TRAUMA)
For mom:
Forgiveness™—Diffuse or apply one to two drops to help release the past.
Present Time™—Diffuse or apply one to two drops to stay focused on the now.
Surrender™—Diffuse or apply one to two drops to support in releasing negative emotions.
Peace & Calming® or Stress Away™ roll on—Apply on wrist and around ears and neck. Rest, relaxation and the ability to think clearly will return. Smelling good will help a mom feel pretty.

ENERGY INCREASE
For mom:
En-R-Gee™—Smell or apply one drop on the back neck, or on bottom of both feet.
NingXia Red®—Drink three to six ounces per day, spread throughout the day. Some people are so energized by **NingXia Red®** that they cannot drink it after 4 p.m.

EPISIOTOMY (also see PERINEUM CARE)
This is a small incision to further open the perineum to allow more room for the baby to be delivered. They often require stitches to aid in healing.
Peace & Calming®—Diffuse during labor.
Lavender—Add several drops to bath water at birth or diffuse it in the room.
LavaDerm™ Cooling Mist—Spray the area after birth.

ClaraDerm™ Spray—Apply as needed for six weeks prior to birth and after to condition and promote healing.

EYE CONDITIONS (clogged tear ducts, pinkeye and sty)
For babies and children:
Lavender—Apply one diluted drop to bridge of the nose and on the bone surrounding the eye, careful to avoid the eye.

For mom:
Lavender—Apply one drop to bridge of the nose and on the bone surrounding the eye, careful to avoid the eye.
Eye support blend:
  Olive Oil (20 drops)
  Lavender (20 drops)
  Melrose™ (20 drops)
  Frankincense (10 drops)
Combine in a small dropper bottle. Place one drop on a clean index finger, rub together with the other index finger. Gently apply around the boney part of the eye. May also be placed on the toe reflex point.

FEAR (also see EMOTIONAL SUPPORT)
For babies or children:
Valor®—Apply or roll-on to bottom of feet and diffuse.

For mom:
Valor®, Surrender™ and Believe™—Wear as a perfume and inhale as needed to help with courage and focus and to dispel any fears associated with pregnancy and childbirth.
FEBRILE SEIZURES

> "I used Present Time™ and Surrender™ to help me with my fear to push, and it was amazing how fast Jack came!"
> ~ Beverly

Febrile seizures are convulsions in a child (common between ages nine months and 5 years) triggered by a fever. Ear infections or any cold or viral illness may trigger a febrile seizure. Though these are rarely a sign of a more serious illness, seek medical attention to rule out anything serious.

Lavender and frankincense—Apply on the head and big toe.

Lemon, melaleuca ericifolia or mountain savory—A few drops diluted on the spine and bottom of feet to combat the virus.

FEVER

If fever persists or begins to rise, seek medical attention.

For babies:

Lavender—Apply one or two drops to the bottom of the feet.

Lemon (diluted 1:30 with carrier oil)—Apply one or two drops to the bottom of the feet and spine.

For children:

Peppermint—Dilute 1:5 and apply to the navel.

Lavender or Thieves® (diluted 1:5 or more)—Apply one or two drops or either to the bottom of the feet hourly.

Lemon (diluted 1:5 with carrier oil)—Apply one or two drops to the bottom of the feet and spine.

NingXia Red®—one ounce every couple of hours.

For mom, same as child plus:

Inner Defense™—one capsule or more daily.

"I found that peppermint brought my daughter Bella's fever down within minutes (as compared to half and hour with Tylenol), and then I used mountain savory on her spine anytime she started to act like she was feeling bad. She was the only one I fought a fever with. So anytime she started to act sick I would put peppermint on her belly button and mountain savory on her spine. She ended up having three seizures total and all those were before I figured out the peppermint thing — she never had another one after that one. One day, she started to have one (eyes glazing over), and I applied the peppermint (knowing the Tylenol would take too long anyway) — I think we timed about three minutes for the fever to start coming down and her eyes to brighten. ~ Beverly

FORMULA ENHANCERS

Many moms are faced with a dilemma: either their milk supply is not sufficient for the baby (even after using the milk-boosting suggestions on page 71) or they are not breast feeding and want to supplement traditional formula. The following enhancers are not to be used in lieu of regular formula but may be used with breastfeeding or with regular formula, especially when milk supply is low or the baby is not gaining weight properly. Consult babies healthcare provider before adding to babies diet.

Enhancer recipe:
    Six ounces of purified water
    One half scoop of **Power Meal** (amino acid and nutrient rich powder)
    One half scoop of **Pure Protein Complete™** (whey-based powder that contains 13 grams of protein per serving)
    One teaspoon to one tablespoon **NingXia Red®**
Mix well in a blender. This also may be mixed with goats milk or rice milk. May adjust amount depending on dietary needs of the child.

FUNGAL INFECTIONS

These may appear on the skin, between toes or folds of skin.

For babies:
Melrose™—Apply one drop diluted on the area.

For mom:
Athletes foot ointment—Use the ingredients below and follow the instructions on page 32 to create this ointment. Apply to clean feet and toes twice daily.
    Abundance™ (two drops)
    Melrose™ (two drops)
    Thieves® (one drop)
    Female Salve—Use the ingredients below and follow the instructions on page 32 to create this ointment. It may be used topically or as an insertion when pregnant or nursing for itching, genital herpes, candida and infections.
    Gentle Baby™ (three drops)

3 Wise Men™ (three drops)
Patchouli (three drops)

⒢ESTATIONAL DIABETES (also see NUTRITION GUIDE on page 88)

This refers to pregnant women who have never had diabetes, but whose blood sugar levels rise during pregnancy. As the baby develops hormones from the placenta, this can block the action of the mother's insulin in her body and make it hard for the mother's body to use insulin. This condition requires monitoring by a health professional to avoid serious complications for mom and baby. Avoid highly processed food, especially refined white flour and white sugar foods. The following may be helpful. Use only if approved by healthcare provider.

NingXia Red®—Three ounces over the course of a day.
Pure Protein Complete™ **or Power Meal**—One to two servings per day between meals.
Ocotea—Two drops in ½ ounce **NingXia Red**® in the morning, mid afternoon and before bedtime.
For a healthy snack, make the green smoothie on page 91.

I tested positive for gestational diabetes with my first child and then again with my fourth. I managed to control it with diet during my first pregnancy. However, with my fourth, I was so frustrated and had to almost starve myself to keep my sugars down. I was absolutely fearful that I would have to go on insulin. Then I got my NingXia Red®. I started taking one ounce three times a day, following each meal. Within three to four days, I noticed a dramatic difference. My sugars were less than 120 almost all the time. I was usually high once or twice a week after starting NingXia Red®, but when I was high, it was only in the 130s not the 180s. After a week, I noticed that I was able to eat larger portions and still maintain my sugars within range. That is awesome when you are pregnant and hungry almost all the time! I had a healthy, full-term, eight pound baby girl with zero complications. Praise God! ~ Becky, R.N.

GROUP BETA STREP

The bacteria Group B Streptococcus (GBS) has been identified as the number one cause of life-threatening infections in newborns. Normally found in 40 percent of all healthy women, those who test positive for GBS are said to be colonized. This should not be confused with Group A Streptococcus, which causes strep throat. Please consult your healthcare provider. Treatment may require antibiotics.

To reduce risk:

Thieves®—Apply three drops on soles of feet morning and night.
Valor®—Apply five drops distributed along the spine, morning and night.
Inner Defense™—Three to five capsules daily. See testimony in back of book.
Life 5™ Probiotic—One capsule each evening.

HAND-FOOT-AND-MOUTH DISEASE

This is a common childhood illness which may feature mouth sores, fever and a rash. It may be caused by a variety of viruses in the Enterovirus family, specifically coxsackievirus A16. This condition is not to be confused with foot and mouth disease, which infects cattle and is rare in humans.

Melrose™, Purification®, lavender, Thieves®*, mountain savory—Dilute or apply two or three drops neat on the feet and spine several times throughout the day. These oils also may be alternated. *Thieves® contains several ingredients listed as cautionary and may be omitted if concerned.

A few days before we were going out of town to see family, I noticed red bumps/blisters on my son's feet. Because he had slept terribly the night before, I immediately suspected hand-foot-and-mouth disease. He did not have blisters on his hands or mouth, nor did he have a fever or other symptoms. I chalked it up to teething. By lunchtime, he had developed the blisters on his hands. I still didn't see any in his mouth, but I knew it had to be the virus especially when he wouldn't eat solids for dinner that night. I began to apply Thieves® on his feet and spine. I alternated with mountain savory and Purification®. Just an hour or so after applying the Purification®, I tried to show the bumps to my mom, and I could only find two! I kept applying the Purification® at every diaper change on Monday and continued as we traveled Tuesday. By Wednesday, the bumps we gone from his hands and only red spots remained on his feet! He never seemed to have the fever, but the Purification® really seemed to have shortened the duration of the virus! ~ Wendy

HEADACHES
For mom:
Lavender—Place a drop on temples, back of neck, across forehead and on the painful location. Also inhale.
Frankincense—Place a drop on temples, back of neck, across forehead and on the painful location. Also inhale.
Peppermint—Place a drop on temples, back of neck, across forehead and where discomfort exists. Also inhale. **Peppermint** may cause a reduction in milk supply if nursing, and some aromatherapy texts suggest avoiding during pregnancy.
Roman Chamomile—Place a drop or less on temples, back of neck, and across forehead where discomfort exists. Also inhale.

HEART BURN (see also ACID REFLUX)
For babies, SEE COLIC.
Mom:
Copaiba—Ingest one drop or apply one to two drops on the chest when needed.
DiGize™—Apply three to four drops directly on the mother's belly. May also ingest one drop orally.
A combination of the above works best.
NingXia Red®—Sip on as needed.
AlkaLime®—Dissolve one teaspoon in four ounces of water and drink early morning and late evening.

HEMORRHOIDS

Rose Ointment™—Apply topically.

Balance Complete™—Eat plenty of nutritious fiber. **Balance Complete™** is a great high-fiber, high-protein, nutritionally dense drink mix and is delicious in smoothies.

Hemorrhoid Relief Blend—Combine the following oils with two to four drops of V-6™ oil and apply to the area.

Peppermint (one drop)
Helichrysum (two drops)
Geranium (two drops)
Cypress (two drops)

Hemorrhoid ointment #1—Use the ingredients below and follow the instructions on page 32 to create this ointment. Apply until problem solved.

Cypress (three drops)
Cistus (two drops)
Basil (three drops)
Spikenard (one drop)
Wintergreen (one drop)

Hemorrhoid ointment #2—Use the ingredients below and follow the instructions on page 32 to create this ointment. Apply until problem solved.

Cypress (four drops)
Myrtle (two drops)
Myrrh (two drops)
Roman Chamomile (two drops)

"After Jack's birth, I had a hemorrhoid that was very uncomfortable. I tried all the normal stuff — more fiber, water, etc. — and just could not get it to go away. Finally, I put together this blend of one drop peppermint, two drops helichrysum, and two drops cypress, and a couple drops of V-6™ oil. In less than a week it was completely gone!"
~ Beverly

INDIGESTION
For babies and children:
Lemon or copaiba—Apply a drop on the bottom of the feet diluted 1:10.

For mom:
Peppermint, lemon or copaiba—Place one drop on the tongue.
Peppermint may cause a reduction in milk supply if nursing and some aromatherapy texts suggest avoiding during pregnancy.
AlkaLime®—Put one teaspoon in water in the morning and evening on an empty stomach, may take after a meal if indigestion is severe.
Essentialzyme™—Two tablets with a meal to aid in digestion.

INSECT BITES
Roman Chamomile or Purification®—Apply one drop on a bite. Repeat every 15 minutes as needed for swelling or itching.
Insect Repellent Spray—Gentle enough for babies. For every four ounces of distilled water add five drops of **Purification®** and five drops of **peppermint**, **palo santo** (bed bugs), **Idaho tansy** (flies) in a spray bottle. Lightly spray the clothing before going outside. May also spray exposed arms and legs.

"I have a few kids that swell up immediately with any kind of insect bite. Just a dab of Purification® oil, and the bites are gone within minutes." ~ Jeanette

"During the late summer and early fall, I put Purification® on my newborn daughter's feet every day to combat any germs my husband, a teacher and coach, might bring home. The baby stayed healthy, and, as an added benefit, I noticed that neither she nor I had the usual mosquito bites that were possible year round in South Texas." ~ Laura

INSOMNIA—Mom
Lavender and Peace & Calming®—Apply two drops each to the bottom of the feet at bedtime. May also diffuse in the bedroom 30 minutes before retiring.

ITCHING (also see SKIN and FUNGAL INFECTIONS)
For mom:
Rose or geranium and Roman chamomile—Place one drop of each into a ½ tsp. of salt and add to the bath water to make a Sitz bath.

Rose Ointment™—Apply to area.
LavaDerm™ Cooling Mist—Spray on area.
ClaraDerm™ Spray—Spray on area.
Roman Chamomile—Apply topically and may be combined with **Rose Ointment™**.

JAUNDICE
This occurs when abnormally high levels of the bile pigment, also known as bilirubin, in the blood stream can cause the yellow discoloration of the skin and whites of the eyes. Consult healthcare provider.
Lemon, geranium or orange oil—Place one drop of either oil diluted with two drops carrier oil applied to the bottom of the feet 2-3 times daily.
Place the baby near a window or go out for a walk in order to get 10 minutes of indirect sunlight daily. A mother's good diet, while pregnant and during frequent nursing, generally will abate newborn jaundice within a few days.

LABOR AND DELIVERY
Please note that as with many suggestions, mothers must take a 'wait and see' approach for the desired results. The amount of oil needed may vary from case to case depending on a mother's prior experiences. All of these oils can be diffused, directly inhaled or added to bath water (two to four drops).

To halt EARLY labor:
Lavender—Apply a few drops on the belly to help calm and relax mom.
Peace & Calming®—Apply one drop on the heart and solar plexus (chest), or diffuse.

Encourage labor:
Jasmine—Apply as a perfume or inhale once labor begins. Do not use internally.

During labor:
Labor Blend—Mix the following oils with ½ ounce of V-6™ oil for use only after the labor starts. Massage two to four drops of the mixture inside the ankles, on little toes, little fingers, lower abdomen and back.
  Helichrysum (four drops)
  Fennel (four drops)
  Peppermint (two drops)
  Ylang Ylang (six drops)
  Clary Sage (three drops)
Frankincense—Dilute 1:1 and apply around vaginal opening.
Valor®—Apply four to six drops on wrists, chest, back of neck and/ or bottom of the feet. Wait five to 10 minutes before applying another oil. Also, diffuse one to two drops on chest, back of neck and base of spine during transitional labor/pushing.
Peace & Calming®—Apply a drop to wrists, edge of ears and/or bottom of feet.
Brain Power™—Apply one to two drops on neck, throat, temples and/or under nose.
En-R-Gee™—Apply along the spine and/or one to two drops to wrists, temples, back of neck, behind ears or feet.
Ylang Ylang—Apply one to two drops of either or both on Vita Flex points on feet to advance labor.
Diffusing blend
  Lavender (4 drops)
  Frankincense (4 drops)
  Ylang Ylang (2 drops)
  Roman Chamomile (2 drops)
Diffuse in birthing room. Adjust amounts according to diffuser.
Washcloth blend—Place the following oils in a bowl of water, swish a washcloth in it and use it to cool mom's head and face.
  Jasmine (5-10 drops)
  Roman Chamomile (5 drops)

Geranium (5 drops)
Lavender (10-20 drops)
Afterbirth blend—Use the following oils with a carrier oil on the abdomen to help expel placenta and tone the uterus.
Geranium (5-10 drops)
Lavender (5-10 drops)
Jasmine (7-15 drops)

"Having used my YL oils, I felt so relaxed that it only took three swift pushes and our baby girl came only one hour and 10 minutes after arriving at the hospital. My precious husband called me 'Superwoman' because I got up out of the labor and delivery bed and walked to my private room on the other side of the hospital. That's how relaxed yet revitalized I felt. The nurses were dumbfounded and in awe. The oils really kept me relaxed and focused!" ~ Karen

"We had our baby after only one hour and 33 minute labor. I arrived at the hospital door only eight minutes before she was here. Thank you for all of the advise and support through *Gentle Babies* during this pregnancy. It has helped a lot to know that I had alternatives to modern medicine when facing certain issues. NingXia Red® was invaluable throughout this pregnancy!" ~ Neisha

"I loved having the oils during my labor and delivery! Peace & Calming® was my favorite and helped me relax. I was so excited to be able to anoint my baby with oils right after his birth. We sprayed ClaraDerm™ with frankincense, myrrh, lavender and helichrysum on our hands to anoint his head and then sprayed directly all over his body and on the umbilical cord area. My baby's skin was so smooth and soft, and he smelled great! After the birth, I loved knowing that all of the oils I used would also kill any potential bacteria or viruses in the environment around us." ~ Sera

LACTATION
To increase:
Fennel—Swallow two drops of the oil in a teaspoon of honey every two hours. Follow with a glass of water. May apply to breast following a nursing session. Avoid if a family history of seizures exists.
Joy™, Stress Away™—Inhale to help calm and soothe as stress may have negative interference with lactation.
Prepare and enjoy the green smoothie on page 91.

To decrease:
Clary Sage—Ingest two drops and apply neat to each breast two or three times per day.
Peppermint—Five drops orally several times per day. *Most herbal books will suggest avoiding **peppermint** during nursing as it may decrease milk supply; however, many mothers who have used **peppermint** report that it did not effect their lactation.

"I have lost my milk around six or eight months with every child I have had. With my fourth, I began losing it at five months. I read about using fennel and began putting a drop in my water bottle each day and rubbing it on my chest. I saw results within a few hours, and my milk supply is increasing. After Jack did not nurse for two days due to congestion, my milk supply was low. I take one drop of fennel under the tongue and rub a drop or two across the chest, and my milk supply has visibly increased." ~ Beverly

"A lactation consultant determined the breastfeeding issues my daughter, Shula, had were because I was producing way too much milk, causing my letdown to be too strong. Pumping off the excess milk would be a temporary fix, as my brain still would be triggered to keep producing an overabundance of milk. My breasts had become painfully engorged with hard lumps in each of them, and my daughter fed for such short periods of time that there was no relief. I took two drops of clary sage orally and rubbed

two drops neat per breast twice the first day and three times the second day to decrease my milk supply. Also, I would hand-express milk for 20 to 30 seconds before each feeding to soften the areola and slow the ejection force without stimulating my brain to produce more milk. Lastly, I fed Shula every three hours and stayed on the same breast for two to three feedings in a row. By the third day, my painful lumps and engorgement had disappeared, and my milk supply was in a much more manageable range."
~ Shannon

MASSAGE
See page 29 for detailed information about infant massage.

MORNING SICKNESS (also see NAUSEA & VOMITING)
Homemade herbal tea for morning sickness:
   1 teaspoon cloves
   1 teaspoon Turkey Rhubarb herb
   1 teaspoon cinnamon
   1 ounce fresh or dried spearmint
Simmer the first three herbs in one pint of water for five minutes. Pour this decoction over the spearmint in a glass jar and secure the lid. Let infuse until cool or twenty minutes, then strain. Take two tablespoons to ¼ cup every hour until nausea subsides. *(Provided by Sandra Ellis, M.H.)*
Spearmint (two drops), ginger (one drop), and patchouli (one drop)—Combine in a capsule at the onset or to prevent, or inhale and rub over belly.
Progessence™ Plus Serum—a progesterone serum with essential oils. May be used the first few months of pregnancy to aid in balancing hormone levels. Extreme cases — hyperemesis gravid arum — may be the result of very low progesterone. **PD 80/20™** is a supplement many women turn to. Consult your health care provider to see if either is advised.

MOUTHWASH/ORAL HYGIENE

Thieves® Mouthwash—Swish and swallow for fresh breath. If sensitivity to breath smell of labor support team, have them swish and swallow.

Peppermint, spearmint, orange or lemon oil—Apply a drop of any to the tongue.

MUSCULAR ACHES

Deep Relief, Stress Away™ or Aroma Siez™—Apply as needed to sore muscles with a squirt of V-6™ or other carrier oil.

Ortho Sport Massage Oil—Apply liberally for muscular and skeletal ache.

Marjoram, Idaho balsam fir, copaiba or palo santo—Apply directly on muscles or dilute with carrier oil.

Valor®—Apply directly on sore areas and/or on bottom of feet and/or on spine.

NAUSEA (see the NUTRITION GUIDE on page 88)
For mom:

DiGize™—Rub over the abdomen and put on drop on the finger to the inside of the cheeks. **DiGize™** contains fennel. Avoid if a family history of seizures exists.

Thieves®—Apply a few drops to the feet. Inhale from bottle.

Sandalwood—Rub one to two drops over abdomen.

PD 80/20™—Use as directed after consulting with a health care provider.

Peppermint—Inhale or apply one drop on tongue.

Lemon, orange or tangerine—Mix five drops with a quart of pure water in a glass container and drink throughout the day. Do not put the oil in a plastic container as it may react with petrochemical products.

NingXia Red®—Drink one to two ounces a day in the morning. Homemade herbal tea for morning sickness (see recipe on page 72)

Core Supplements, JuvaPower®, MultiGreens™, Balance Complete™, Mineral Essence™ and NingXia Red®—Use as directed to boost nutrition.

NUTRITION (see DIETARY REGIMEN DURING PREGNANCY and NUTRITION GUIDE on page 88)

*P*ANIC (also see EMOTIONAL SUPPORT)
Stress Away™ or Peace & Calming®—Apply on the body, chest and wrists or diffuse or use in a bath.
Lavender—Same application as above.

PERINEUM CARE (also see EPISIOTOMY PREVENTION)
One month before delivery:
Clary sage (five drops) and rose (two drops)—Mix with one ounce of carrier oil and apply to perineal area.
Myrrh—Dilute 1:10 with carrier oil and apply topically.
ClaraDerm™ Spray—Spray each day or several times a day on the perineum, for the six weeks prior to delivery.

Three weeks before delivery:
Geranium (eight drops) and lavender (five drops)—Mix with one ounce almond oil and rub on the perineum three times a day. This may help to soften the cervix and thin the membrane to get ready for delivery.

One week before delivery:
Geranium (eight drops), lavender (five drops) and fennel (five drops)—Mix with one ounce carrier oil and apply on the perineum to further get it ready.

Perineal massage once labor is established:
Myrrh—Dilute a few drops 1:10 and apply to perineum.

Perineal tear and trauma:
ClaraDerm™ Spray—Apply several times, even hourly, daily.
Melrose™—Dilute 1:10 and apply to perineum
Cypress (two drops) and lavender (three drops)—Add oils to ½ tsp. of salt and mix into bath water to create a Sitz bath.

"I had a small tear with the birth of my fourth child, and ClaraDerm™ Spray was so wonderful and soothing. It even helped heal the tear faster than when I tore with my other children. No new mother should be without their ClaraDerm™." ~ Sera

PINK EYE

Wash hands thoroughly when applying the following ideas:
If lactating: Express ½ ounce breast milk into a sterile cup cooled to room temperature. Use a sanitized dropper and place one to two drops in the affected eye.

Melrose™ and lavender—Place one drop of each with one drop of olive oil onto a clean, sterile plate. Mix together. Use a scant amount of oil on finger to massage the outer bone of the eye socket, bridge of the nose, above the eye brow and the temple. There should be little to no oil residue on the skin after massaging. Be sure to use a small amount and avoid getting it into baby's eye. Nap time and night time are good times to use this formula. Cover the plate or bowl and reuse the formula twice per day; this is enough for several applications. *These essential oils, when used as directed, yield great results. Although a YL essential oil accidentally placed in the eye will not damage the eye, it may agitate it temporarily. If this occurs, put a few drops of V-6™ oils to dilute it, and the agitation should cease immediately. Do not use water.

PLACENTA PREVIA

Placenta previa is a pregnancy complication in which the placenta has attached to the uterine wall close to or covering the cervix. If you experience painless bright red bleeding, be sure to contact your health care provider immediately. Please see your healthcare provider as this can be a serious concern in pregnancy and requires monitoring.

POISON IVY
For child:
KidScents® MightyZymes—Take tablets between meals (up to eight per day) as directed on bottle.

For mom:
ClaraDerm™ Spray—Spray on the affected area, repeat hourly until the condition is resolved.

POSTPARTUM DEPRESSION (also see EMOTIONAL SUPPORT)
This may arrive with onset of lactation, one to four days after birth.
Thyromin™—Two to three capsules at night to support thyroid gland function.
Jasmine—Add a few drops to ½ tsp. of salt and mix into bath water. **Ylang ylang** or **clary sage** may be substituted for **Jasmine**.
Rose or Joy™ or Idaho balsam fir—Inhale and wear daily as a perfume.
Frankincense—Diffuse or apply anywhere on the body, direct or diluted 1:1.
Bergamot (two drops), ylang ylang (two drops) and clary sage (two drops)—Add to ½ teaspoon of salt and mix into bath water.
Feelings Kit—Use as directed or desired.
Progessence™ Plus Serum—Use as directed on bottle with healthcare provider approval.

PREECLAMPSIA (see page 45)

PRENATAL VITAMINS (see VITAMINS)

"Instead of taking over-the-counter prenatal vitamins, I chose with great confidence to take Master Formula HERS™."
~ Karen

"My favorite prenatal vitamin regimen was Core Supplements, extra Omega Blue™ (now known as OmegaGize³™) and NingXia Red®. I felt great!" ~ Sera

PUBIS DIASTIS
This is an abnormally wide gap between the two pubic bones and can be very painful. To ease discomfort:
Rose Ointment™ and Idaho balsam fir—Apply one or two drops of oil with the ointment and apply over the pubic area to relieve discomfort.
BLM™—Two to four capsules daily as directed on the bottle for bone health support.

RESPIRATORY INFECTION (also see COUGHING and CONGESTION)
Consult you healthcare provider if coughing persists or the child has difficulty breathing.
For baby:
Myrtle, Idaho balsam, copaiba, frankincense or ravintsara—Dilute 1:1 or more to the baby's feet or back of chest. Cover with undershirt.
Peace & Calming®—Dilute 1:30 and apply to chest area to calm a cough.

"When my son Caleb was just three months old, he came down with what seemed to be a very bad cold. He was very stuffy and miserable and couldn't sleep. The next day the pediatrician tested him, and Caleb was positive for RSV. Since my mother and husband had just been sick with bad respiratory infections that traveled to their chests, the doctor said the same would happen to Caleb. In addition, RSV makes some babies' oxygen levels drop so that they have to go to the emergency room, and I just could not let that happen. My friend, Sera, came over and brought her RSV blend of Thieves®, oregano, Raven™ and R.C.™ We applied it to Caleb's feet and diffused Thieves® all day. He was still a little stuffy that night, but, by the next day, he was almost all clear, and, by the third day, all signs of infection were gone! After that, I was hooked and have been using essential oils with my family ever since." ~ Wendy

For mom:
Myrtle, ravintsara, peppermint, R.C.™, Thieves® or frankincense—Dilute 1:1 and apply to the feet several times each day as needed. If pregnant, consult your healthcare provider.
Inner Defense™—Take as directed on bottle.

RINGWORM
Melrose™—Apply diluted or neat depending on age of child to area of concern.
Thieves® Household Cleaner—Clean everything including bedding and clothing to prevent the spread.

ROSACEA (also see SKIN)
Frequently appearing on the face, eyelids, elbows and back, Rosacea, also known as adult acne, may take both internal cleansing and external essential oils to provide complete relief.
Lavender Hand & Body Lotion—Apply to the affected area two to three times each day until resolved.

SANITIZING
Thieves® Household Cleaner may be diluted to various strengths for cleaning the whole house including babies room, toys, laundry and changing table. See House Cleaning on page 35.

SELF-ESTEEM (also see EMOTIONAL SUPPORT)
Believe™—Apply as perfume, directly or diluted.
Valor®—Apply on the soles of the feet or a drop on the chest.

SELF-LOVE (also see EMOTIONAL SUPPORT)
For those days when mom may be feeling down:
Rose—Apply one drop over heart.
Joy™ and Present Time™—Apply one drop of either or both as perfume on wrists and inhale.
Feelings Kit—Use as directed or desired.

SKIN—DRY
For baby:
Rose—Dilute 1:30 with carrier oil and apply to skin.
Rose Ointment™—Apply to dry spots.
KidScents® Lotion—Apply to entire body.
Animal Scents™ Ointment—Apply to the affected area.

"During pregnancy, I keep a bottle of Gentle Baby™ and KidScents® Tender Tush in the shower. When I am done with my hot shower, I turn the water off and apply both to my belly — I did not have any 'extra' stretch marks this pregnancy. Wish I would have known this with my first three." ~ Beverly

"As my tummy began to get larger, I applied a homemade salve night and day to keep it from feeling so dry and itchy. The salve, which is made with YL essential oils, started removing old stretch marks and kept new ones from appearing. I had the prettiest baby belly I had ever seen. I could have been in a magazine without touchups." ~ Karen

"All of my life I have dealt with psoriasis which is a very complex issue encompassing diet, enzymes, candida, digestive health and even emotional health. The first thing I did to address the psoriasis, was to get rid of all of the toxins in my home — from my personal care products to household cleaners — and switch to the Young Living brand for toothpastes, soaps, shower gels, shampoos, conditioners and Thieves® household cleaner. I also improved my diet, began drinking NingXia Red® daily, cleansed and supplemented with Core Complete and a daily intake of essential oils. Three and a half years later, I found the psoriasis to ease up a bit ever so slightly around my body. In the Spring of 2009, I started using the new Lavender Hand & Body Lotion. After about a month or two of using this lotion, I realized the worst patch — on my left elbow — was totally gone as were the patches on my hands and feet!" ~ Sera

For mom:
Genesis™ Lotion—Apply to the entire body.
Mom's Skin Delight Blend—For itchy skin. Combine the following ingredients and apply the mixture as often as each day to wet skin after showering, especially on the growing belly. It may help soothe itching and could be beneficial for stretch marks too. May be best to find the root cause and address it for full recovery.

2½ tablespoons of almond oil
½ tablespoon jojoba oil
One Evening Primrose capsule (approximately 10 drops)
One Vitamin E capsule (approximately 10 drops)
Tangerine oil (four drops)
Geranium (four drops)
Lavender (four drops)
Cypress (four drops)
Lemon oil (three drops)

Drops of Gold Facial Blend—Use the ingredients listed below to create this blend. Apply to the face, neck and arms for radiant and healthy looking skin. Recipe may be reduced for smaller quantities but is best if bottled in 1/2 ounce bottles. Recipe may be adjusted according to the amount you wish to make.

Two ounces almond oil
One ounce jojoba oil
Two ounces Evening Primrose oil
Vitamin E oil (40 drops)
Patchouli (48 drops)
Frankincense (40 drops)
Geranium (24 drops)
Palmarosa (16 drops)
Lavender (16 drops)
Rose (5 drops)

SLEEPLESSNESS
For babies and children:
Cedarwood or Peace & Calming®—Dilute 1:2 and apply on soles of feet at nap time or bedtime. Also may diffuse 20 to 30 minutes in the bedroom before bed.

Lavender—Same application as above and apply a drop on the pillow or put in bath water.

Valor®—When **Peace & Calming®** does not help, apply on soles of feet before bedtime.

Tranquil™ Roll-On—Apply to back of the neck, soles of the feet and wrists. Also inhale.

SORE NIPPLES

Rose—Mix one or two drops in five ounces of sweet almond oil or V-6™ oil.

Rose Ointment™—Apply topically as needed.

Nursing Mom's Best Friend Ointment—Use the ingredients below and follow the instructions on page 32 to create this ointment. Apply to dry, cracked nipples after nursing and wipe clean before nursing to avoid a bad taste in baby's mouth.

   Geranium (four drops)
   St. Maries Lavender (two drops)
   Myrrh (two drops)
   Gentle Baby™ (two drops)

SORE THROATS
For babies:
Melaleuca ericifolia, lemon and/or lavender—Apply diluted to bottom of feet and diffuse a short time in babies room.

For children over five years old:
Thieves® and oregano—Apply diluted or neat on the bottoms of the feet three times per day.

Melaleuca ericifolia, lemon, lavender, palo santo or frankincense—Apply one drop over the throat. May dilute to distribute evenly with carrier oil or lotion.

For children over age five: may use the above or:
NingXia Red®—Freeze the one-ounce single packets frozen and serve as popsicles.

Thieves® Mouthwash—Gargle two to three times per day. Pour into a spray bottle to spray once to the back of the throat. This may be a little hot at first but will be soothing and fight infection. Repeat as needed.

Thieves® Mouthwash—Use as directed.

For mom, may use the above or:
Thieves® Hard Lozenges—Use as directed.
Super C™—Follow bottle instruction for use.
NingXia Red®—Drink slowly throughout the day.

STRETCH MARKS

For best results, rotate these oil/blend treatments.

PREVENTION:
KidScents® Tender Tush—Apply topically a few times per day. It may be applied with **Gentle Baby™** after bathing.
Lavender—Mix one or two drops with V-6™ oil.
Gentle Baby™—Mix one or two drops with V-6™ oil or mix two to four drops with **Rose Ointment™** over abdomen.
Valor®—Apply a few drops neat.

SOLUTION FOR OLD STRETCH MARKS:
Continue prevention protocol.
Gentle Baby™ and Prenolone®+Body Cream—Apply topically each day after bathing.

TEETHING
For baby:
Orange, frankincense or copaiba—Dilute 1:30 and apply directly to affected area.
Exodus II™—Apply one drop diluted 1:30 several times per day to relieve discomfort.

For children:
Clove or Thieves®—Dilute 1:5 with V-6™ oil and massage the baby's gum and tooth area.
PanAway® or Deep Relief—Apply neat to the jaw over the area in pain.

"As one of my daughter's molars came in, it had a large pocket of fluid over it and the gum. She was in pain and had diarrhea. I applied a drop of Exodus II™ several times a day for pain relief. Within two days, the pocket disappeared, and the tooth started to come through. Now she brings me the oils when she wants to taste or 'wear' them." ~ Laura

THRUSH (see also FUNGAL INFECTIONS)
Nursing mothers may experience an outbreak of candida in the form of an infection appearing in creamy white, slightly raised lesions stemming from the overuse of antibiotics. In addition, certain illnesses and stress can disturb the delicate balance of the body.

For baby:
NingXia Red®—Dip a small amount on a clean finger and swab baby's mouth before nursing.
Geranium, lavender, melaleuca ericafilia or Melrose™—Place only a scant amount on a clean finger and swab the baby's mouth. After a few minutes, nurse to remove the taste.

For mom:
NingXia Red®—Nursing moms may drink one to three ounces daily. Dip a small amount on a clean finger and swab baby's mouth several times per day.
Life 5™ Probiotic—One to two capsules daily to replenish lost intestinal flora.

TIREDNESS (also see ENERGY)
For mom: (not when pregnant)
Rosemary—Mix 10 drops in a teaspoon of Epsom salt and add to the bath water.
Orange oil (six drops) and geranium (two drops)—Mix these oils with two tablespoons of V-6™ oil for an invigorating massage oil blend to apply topically as needed.
En-R-Gee™ oil—smell, wear or use in massage.

TRAUMA (also see EMOTIONAL SUPPORT and PERINEUM TEAR)

Trauma Life™—Dilute 1:30 with carrier and apply to the mother after birth to combat physical and psycho-emotional trauma. Maybe applied wherever mom desires or on the back and feet after birth.

UMBILICAL CORD

Myrrh—Dilute 1:10 with carrier oil and apply to the end of the umbilical cord for better healing.

Frankincense—Apply one to two drops per day directly on the umbilical cord stump until it falls off, generally in one week.

Geranium—Apply one to two drops for any bleeding around the umbilical cord/belly button. This may be diluted.

Rose Ointment™ or Animal Scents™ Ointment—apply to area to promote healing.

Umbilical cord ointment—Use the ingredients below and follow the instructions on page 32 to create this ointment. Apply topically until healed. To make a ¼ ounce portion, usually all that is needed, use:

    Lavender (one drop)
    Frankincense (one drop)
    Myrrh (one drop)

URINARY TRACT INFECTION (UTI)

For pregnant mom: (Consult healthcare provider for use of essential oils orally while pregnant)

Lemon or Idaho balsam fir—very powerful in eliminating infection, two to 10 drops in a capsule twice daily. May be applied over bladder

Melrose™—Apply neat over bladder area.

Cranberry—Eat unsweetened, dried or fresh cranberries or drink unsweetened cranberry juice daily throughout the course of a day. Cranberry capsules also may be taken as directed. Because cranberries can be drying to the bladder and kidneys, do not take for prolonged periods. Blueberry juice is an alternative for those who do not like the tartness of cranberry juice.

WATER RETENTION (see EDEMA)

WHOOPING COUGH (also see COUGHING and RESPIRATORY INFECTION)
Roman Chamomile—Diffuse several drops about 15 to 20 minutes throughout the day. If a diffuser is not available, put three drops in hot water and place a safe distance from baby. This allows the baby to smell the vapors.

YEAST INFECTIONS (see also THRUSH)
An infection caused by strains of candida, especially candida albicans, that generally resides in the intestinal tract. This overgrowth may be present in the mucous membranes of the mouth and vagina.

For baby:
NingXia Red®—Dip a small amount on a clean finger and swab baby's mouth before nursing.
Geranium, lavender, melaleuca ericafilia or Melrose™—Place only a scant amount on a clean finger and swab the baby's mouth. After a few minutes, nurse to remove the taste.
Melrose™—Apply diluted 1:30 or neat to the lower abdomen.

For mom:
Mountain Savory—Three to five drops taken orally, two times per day. (University of Montpellier, 1970, "highly effective against yeast and candida".)
Life 5™ Probiotic—One capsule in the evening after dinner. One in the morning if infection is widespread.
Inner Defense™—Take as directed on the bottle.
Vaginal suppository—Do not use while pregnant. In a coconut oil base, combine **mountain savory** (2 drops), **myrtle** (2 drops), **frankincense** (2 drops). Use nightly for two weeks.

As of this edition, YL has introduced a KidScents® Collection of oils suitable for use with small children. We would love to hear your experiences with these oils and include them in the next edition.

Nutrition Guide

"Who satisfies thy mouth with good things, so that thy youth is renewed like the eagle's." Psalm 103:5

Nutrition should take center stage in an expectant or nursing mother's life. It is critical to stay healthy and deliver the growing baby all the nutrition needed for him or her to be a healthy child. Making necessary changes to the family diet now will have long-term, positive habit-forming benefits. Here are some guidelines to follow while pregnant.

In general, opt for more homemade meals with an abundance of raw fruits and vegetables, whole grains, nuts, seeds, sprouts and quality protein. Some moms, especially as the pregnancy progresses, will find eating smaller meals more often is a better choice. Beware of spicy, greasy foods that are not nutrient dense and can be difficult to digest. Spicy foods also can upset the stomach of a nursing baby.

Most health professionals will agree that a daily multiple vitamin is in order. My choice is True Source™, or the complete Core Supplements from Young Living Essential Oils; these are all-natural, food-based nutriceuticals. A great addition to mom's diet is a green drink to include extra vegetables for added nutrition. JuvaPower®, a powder added to water or juice, mixed in with foods, and/or sprinkled on vegetables and in salads is delicious.

Nursing is not the time to go on a diet to drop extra pounds gained while pregnant; nursing naturally helps the body shed those pounds. Moms who eat nutritiously while nursing are more likely to normalize their weight and have happy, healthy babies.

VEGETABLES

Consuming a large quantity of raw and lightly steamed vegetables gives the body loads of nutrition. Select a wide variety and make a big salad topped with legumes (beans) or lean protein part of the daily menu. Dark green leafy vegetables are good sources of calcium and iron. Include the enzyme blend Essentialzyme™ or the chewable KidScents® MightyZymes if gas or bloating are an issue.

FRUITS

When consuming fruits, raw is best and in small amounts. The natural sugar from fruits can raise blood sugar levels for some individuals. A good afternoon snack may include a serving of fruit with nuts or nut butter (See recipe below under Nuts and Seeds). Fruit also makes good dessert options rather than high sugar cakes and cookies.

GRAINS

Avoid refined and over-processed foods, such as white flour, white sugar and boxed meals full of low-quality and unknown ingredients. Select whole grain breads and pastas for their higher nutritional value and low glycemic index. Grains comprise the largest carbohydrate category; some carbohydrates can raise blood sugar levels as much as, or more, than sugar. Elevated blood sugar levels can lead to gestational diabetes. The doctor or midwife will check for this and make necessary recommendations.

NUTS AND SEEDS

Nuts and seeds are full of good fats that both mom and baby need. If digesting them is difficult, use them as nut butter on toast or bread. Available in many varieties, nuts also are a good source of protein and may be consumed raw or cooked/roasted. To make a truly delicious nut butter, put two cups of assorted nuts in a food processor or powerful blender and process until smooth and creamy. No additional salt or oils are required, and the taste is superb. Currently, there is much controversy over eating raw nuts and seeds. Although many believe eating them raw is more nutritious, an expectant mother should consult with her doctor or midwife.

PROTEIN

Turkey, chicken, lean beef, fish and eggs comprise the recommended animal protein. Legumes, nuts, grains and seeds provide non-animal protein. Buckwheat is the king of plant proteins and is easily added to baked goods and also found in cereals.

DAIRY

Plenty of calcium can be obtained from dark green, leafy vegetables, but many moms feel the need to consume milk. Milk can be mucous forming and constipating, but, if mom must have milk, the best choice is organic raw milk from a trusted source. There also is much controversy over raw milk, and it is illegal to purchase it in some states.

FATS

Other than cold-pressed oils, such as olive, sunflower and flax, avoid consuming hydrogenated fats. Fried food is not beneficial to either mom or baby while pregnant or nursing.

FIBER

It is generally recommended that women eat 25 to 30 grams of fiber daily. Fiber can be found in whole grains, vegetables and fruits. A serving of whole grains at each meal will help mom achieve the recommended amounts. Fiber is important for proper bowel function. One serving of delicious Balance Complete™ contains 11 grams of fiber and is a great in-between meal snack or a breakfast meal on the go.

SUGARS

Always avoid foods rich in white, refined sugar, including cakes, cookies, candy, pastries, some cereals and soda. Sugar has no nutritional value, does nothing for the body and can be potentially harmful. Moms who crave sweets can use honey, stevia and YL's Yacon Syrup in moderation.

WATER

Healthy water intake each day is estimated to be half the body weight in ounces. For pregnant moms, six more ounces should be added to avoid dehydration.

GREEN SMOOTHIE

Two tablespoons flaxseed
Two tablespoons chia seed
Two tablespoons sesame seed
One cup cold, clean water
½ cup ice
One medium peeled orange
½ avocado

One cup spinach
One cup or two to three kale
leaves
One scoop of Pure Protein
Complete™ powder (optional)

In a blender, combine two tablespoons of flaxseeds, sesame seed and chia seed and blend until it has the consistency of flour. Turn off the blender and scrape the sides of the blender to loosen the seed flour. Add the rest of the ingredient and blend until creamy. Add more water or fresh juice as desired.

• • • • •

Throughout this book various supplements and nutritional suggestions are mentioned; the Resource Guide is on page 115.

• • • • •

FOR THE ENTIRE FAMILY

For a comprehensive guide to this subject, Growing Healthy Homes offers a six-unit study co-authored by Debra Raybern titled **Nutrition 101: Choose Life!** This family-friendly, Biblically-based program overviews each system of the body and the foods that hinder or nourish development. It includes detailed charts on vitamins, minerals, protein, fiber, fats, fruits and vegetables and healthy recipes in each chapter. It also is used as a curriculum to teach children to love God's food. Order a book, CD, e-book or combination set at GrowingHealthyHomes.com.

Birth Kits

Note: Essential oils and products associated with specific issues mentioned in the Balance Guide should be obtained, in addition to the following suggestions and general birthing supplies. If caution is advised, see in Balance Guide under specific health concern.

BASIC BIRTH KIT

Essential 7 Kit—Includes Joy™, Peace & Calming®, lavender, PanAway®, lemon oil and Purification®.
Valor®—Balances the body physically and emotionally, aids central nervous system relaxation and combats on-going aches and pains.
Gentle Baby™—Helps comfort, soothe and reduce stress during pregnancy; prevents stretch marks and scars; aids prenatal bonding with baby; and prepares perineum for labor.
Clary Sage—Supports labor, balancing of hormones and much more.
Fennel—Supports lactation, digestion and colic.
ClaraDerm™ Spray—Prepares perineum before birth and aids healing after birth.

EXPANDED BIRTH KIT

This includes the Basic Kit plus:
Trauma Life™—Combats any trauma to the mom or baby, physically or emotionally, and balances the brain and nervous system. It is the most comprehensive oil in dealing with trauma and healing tissue.
Myrrh—Softens the perineum during labor, analgesic, anesthetic, heals umbilical cord ending and stretch marks, supports the immune system, spiritually uplifting, stimulates upper brain centers and master glands, similar to frankincense and more.

COMPREHENSIVE BIRTH KIT

This includes the Expanded Birth Kit plus:

Frankincense—Purifies, opens brain function, supports pituitary and pineal gland. It is one of the most holy oils for anointing the newborn. Aids in any type of wound healing, enhances immune function and more.

Rose—Because of its high frequency, it is one of the greatest oils in affecting emotions and physical body. May help with healing trauma, stabilizing of moods especially during postpartum, relaxing, anti-scaring and deepens bonding with baby.

Dr. Mom's Wellness Chest

"But Jesus said, 'Suffer little children, and forbid them not, to come unto me; for of such is the kingdom of heaven.'" Matthew 19:14

These are the most commonly mentioned essential oils in this book. Be prepared with these oils at home and away.

Essential oils and blends included in Young Living's Everyday Oils Kit include:

Lavender—For cuts and scrapes, burns, calming, blocked tear ducts, cradle cap and allergies.

Peppermint—For nausea, stomachaches, constipation, fever, headaches and other aches and pains.

Lemon oil—For coughs, fevers, immune support and pH balancing.

Frankincense—For colds, flu, pneumonia, bacterial and viral infections and the umbilical cord stump.

Thieves®—For viral and bacterial infections; anti-fungal and anti-mold.

PanAway®—For achy muscles and joints, headaches and arthritis.

Peace & Calming®—For relaxation and better sleep.

Valor®—For backaches; anti-viral, anti-bacterial.

Purification®—For insect bites, cuts and scrapes, coughs and bronchitis; anti-viral.

Joy™—For uplifting the mood.

Ravintsara™—For upper respiratory infections and congestion.

Additional Young Living Essential Oil Blends mentioned:

Melrose™—For earaches; anti-viral, anti-bacterial and anti-fungal.

R.C.™—For upper respiratory infections, bronchitis, asthma and congestion.

DiGize™—For stomachaches, stomach viruses, excess mucus and constipation.

Testimonies

"As arrows are in the hand of a mighty man, so are children of one's youth." Psalms 127:4

April Mier, mother to three
I sat staring in unbelief at the positive pregnancy test. "Could it really be true?," I thought to myself. It had been seven years since I had had a baby and three years since I had been pregnant and that pregnancy ended in a miscarriage. And here our family was fostering two little ones. Many thought swirled in my head. I had been using Progessence Plus for a while and then with the added stress of caring for traumatized foster children, I began caring for myself with Young Living's Core Essential Complete which included my vitamins, antioxidants, probiotics and fish oil. I also added Super B to ensure I was nutritionally equipped to handle the extra stress and emotions of fostering, and, within two months, I found myself staring at that positive pregnancy test! Thank you, Lord, for giving me the desires of my heart!

As disbelief turned to excitement and joy, I realized that this pregnancy would be the best out of my previous two because I had my Young Living essential oils and supplements to help me through! My previous pregnancies I dealt with the fear. Fear of my allergies flaring up and having to take medicines, fear of the "dreaded" flu season, and fear of labor and delivery as both of mine had ended with trauma. This time, my hubby and I were able to approach my pregnancy with confidence as we were more educated and equipped with our Young Living Essential Oils!

My elated husband, Charles, helped find an awesome midwife who took me and our newly developing baby into her care. I continued to use the Core Essential Complete as my prenatal vitamins. Balance Complete™ shakes and NingXia Red® were perfect for keeping the tummy happy and blood sugars stable during those initial nauseous weeks when food was unappealing.

I also continued using my Progessence™ Plus for 12 weeks as I had learned from my previous miscarriage that sometimes you can lose a baby due to lack of progesterone. Pure Protein Complete™ added to my smoothies helped me get adequate daily protein intake. I took Essentialzyme™-4 during dinnertime and Detoxzyme® in between to ensure complete digestion and also earlier I had learned that these enzymes kept seasonal Fall allergies and asthma flares away. During my pregnancy when I felt the initial signs and symptoms of an illness come on, I confidently used a drop or two of Thieves® or DiGize™ under my tongue and on bottoms of feet. I LOVED that I didn't have to succumb to the yearly flu season fear mongering. Backaches were nicely cared for with loving hands massaging in a drop of Valor®, PanAway® and Peppermint. No medicines, no worries.

One concern that did appear was a return of a liver/gall bladder issue that I had with my second child — cholestasis. There can be potential risks to baby, and, during my whole pregnancy, I had structured my diet and supplementation to support my gallbladder and liver function. Although I was supremely disappointed that it returned, thank God that it wasn't until the very end of my pregnancy (40 weeks). My midwife worked with us to try and get labor started and we were successful!

My labor and delivery were AMAZING!!! We put some Thieves® in the diffuser to created a sanitary atmosphere. When I felt hot and nauseous, my midwife gave me a washcloth with Peppermint on it. Things went pretty quickly, and Charles and I forgot to use the oils for any other purpose during labor except after baby arrived I began to bleed a lot so I immediately called for Cypress and put a drop over my abdomen and on my radial arteries and that was the end of that! Now to enjoy my brand new baby girl — Grace.

Grace was anointed by her father with a combination of myrrh and frankincense that I had prepared in advance. She was vibrant and strong and continues to be to this day!

The BEST aspect of using my Young Living Oils has been the confidence we have in keeping ourselves healthy and safe. I used to be an anxious mom with a family with chronic health issues, and now I am a confident mom with a healthy family. The biggest health challenge we faced, which really opened my eyes to the power of YLEOs, was when my middle daughter developed Strep at five years old. It had been a chronic issue for her as a baby, and I was not sure if the oils would be enough. However when my five year old refused the antibiotics, I decided to give the oils a try. I checked my Essential Oil Desk Reference and made a capsule with Thieves®, oregano, lemon and frankincense which she figured out how to swallow. I couldn't believe the difference in her within hours! I alternated with several different oils such as thyme and mountain savory in place of oregano in order to give a broad spectrum attack. Although she seemed completely well within eight hours, I continued to give these homemade oil capsules three to four times a day for seven days to ensure the Strep was LONG gone!

I cannot say enough about the power of my Young Living Essential Oils and am so grateful that the Lord led me to them six years ago. We look forward to a continued life and health and healing.

Michelle Weil, mother to four
Having previously used oils for anointing, prayer, relaxation and aromatherapy purposes, it has been common to find oils in every room of our home. Our family has been using YLEOs for nearly four years. Our first experience was with a sample of Raven™, which worked so amazingly fast I knew we wanted our own bottle.

Having purchased the YL Everyday Oils Kit ONLY to have frankincense and myrrh, truth in labeling, and the ability to order wholesale at home, I was amazed when ingesting YL lavender oil became the answer to my prayer to regulate the high blood pressure I was on medication daily for three years. The testimonies continued with psoriasis disappearing in two applications versus worsening over two and a half months with prescription creams. Since that time, our family has been on such a spiritual quest of learning about essential oils in the Bible and how common they were as man's first medicine. When our youngest son began to show food allergies and resulting eczema at four months of age, we were amazed to find the oils (frankincense, lavender and lemon internally) to work great when Zyrtec® and Benadryl® had truly caused him serious problems.

We have used YLEOs for everything we need, from minor cuts and scrapes, rashes, insomnia, hormones, migraine headaches and ear infections to digestive, respiratory, lymphatic, immune concerns and truly life threatening issues. Our children are no longer on medications for hyperactivity, no more antibiotics or prescription drugs, and we have our life and freedom back! We are grateful for YL and for the support system we have in those who choose this way of life. We celebrate and look forward to all that you will experience for your family and friends as you use YL oils, supplements, and products. Blessings abound!

Joni Harrell, mother to three

When my youngest child was 18 months old, he was covered from head to toe in a rash of tiny, red dots. It started out in little patches and slowly spread over the course of two weeks until finally it covered every inch of his body. He had no symptoms with this rash. No itching, no fever, no restless nights, no loss of appetite and no complaints. I was baffled. What it could be?

I treated the rash with several different Young Living essential oils trying to figure out what would cure it. After using lavender, Melrose™, geranium and several others oils I still had no success in ridding my son of his rash. The dots looked a little different after trying the variety oils, but nothing was really working.

Since there were no other symptoms that raised a red flag, I waited a few more days before calling my pediatrician to have him checked out. She determined that his rash was a staph infection. She said STAPH INFECTION! What I thought was panic mode before was nothing compared to the frenzy I was in now. Even in my hysteria, my heart sank. My precious baby was covered in staph. Thoughts flooded my mind. How could this happen? Where did he get this? How did he not have other symptoms?

Once I settled down, I remembered praying over my son a few days back. My prayer was that God would show me what his condition was and how to treat it. The first part had been answered; I knew what the rash was. This flashback of my prayers was happening quickly. After hearing "STAPH", I recalled reading an article about Young Living's R.C.™ oil killing MRSA. I told my very understanding pediatrician about R.C.™ and that I wanted to give it a try. She agreed that I should try it and trusted that if it didn't work I would return to her office. Her instructions were to use the oils and, if I saw ANY improvement within one week, I could continue the use of my natural remedy. I rushed home and doused my baby in R.C.™!! I was amazed! In just a few short hours, his rash was changing. It was as though I was watching the infection die off right in front of my every eyes. I couldn't believe it was working so fast. Relief set in and opened my computer. I overnighted more R.C.™ as well as melaleuca alternifolia.

For the next week, I treated him three times a day both topically and orally. I mixed the R.C.™ and melaleuca with lotion and rubbed him from head to toe. I gave him a bath two times a day with an added mix of coconut oil, R.C.™ and melaleuca. For the oral regiment, I mixed ¼ tsp. coconut oil, ¼ tsp. maple syrup, 3-4 drops of R.C.™ and 2-3 drops of melaleuca in a small glass and administered to him through a medicine dropper. I wanted to treat him orally because I wasn't sure if the staph was systemic or just on his skin. Either way, I knew that having him ingest the oils would take care of anything internally but also speed up the healing process of what I could see externally.

Within three weeks his skin was not only clear of staph, it was completely healed. There was no sign of a rash, and there was no damage to his skin. I was impressed and so was my pediatrician. I knew from my previous experiences with Young Living oils that there had to be something to cure his rash. I just had to be persistent and keep trying. I can't deny that I was frustrated when the first oil I tried didn't work. However, in my continued use of YL's quality oils, I've learned that using one particular oil doesn't work the same in every situation. The body and the diseases it carries respond differently to different oils. Some are better for one situation, while others are better for another.

To sum it up for our staph treatment:

• I used R.C.™ and melaleuca alternifolia
• Apply both oils topically three times a day
• Ingest both oils three times a day (3-4 drops R.C.™ and 2-3 drops melaleuca each time with ¼ tsp. coconut oil and ¼ tsp. pure maple syrup)
• Take a bath with a mixture of coconut oil, R.C.™ and melaleuca two times a day

I did this regimen for two weeks and then slowly cut back the dosage amounts as well as the number of times I administered it daily.

Katherine Grimes-Read, C.N.M., R.N., M.S.N.
I read a testimonial by someone who had used peppermint oil on her abdomen to turn a baby from breech (rear down) to vertex (head down). So I used it on two patients, and it worked on one and the other didn't turn. But the one that didn't turn even went to the hospital to have a version — where they manually turn the baby to vertex position — and it didn't work either. I will continue to use peppermint oil for first line treatment to turn breech babies.

Karen Douglas, mother to four
All of my pregnancies were great, but my first with daily usage of essential oils was by far the best.

Before I became pregnant, nutrition had become an important part of my life as I was using Young Living oils and supplements. At the age of 40, I had my fourth child. Instead of using over-the-counter prenatal vitamins, I chose with great confidence to use YL Master Formula HERS™ Vitamins, which have essential oils infused in them. During this pregnancy, I used Valor® all over my abdomen morning and night, lavender on my feet and Brain Power™ on my head. Also, I never left home without applying Peace & Calming® to my wrists, the edges of my ears and the bottoms of my feet for an overall peaceful day. With prayer, my family and I used whatever oils we felt would assist me at that time and found them especially comforting, relaxing and revitalizing.

On Sunday afternoon, I started having mild contractions. My husband Chris began rubbing Valor®, lavender, Brain Power™ and Peace & Calming® on me. He repeated the process again at bedtime. I awoke at 1:30 a.m. Monday morning with strong contractions. At 2:45 a.m. with the oils in hand, we were off to the hospital. I was four centimeters dilated when I arrived at 3 a.m. From the time I arrived and was taken to my labor and delivery room, 45 minutes passed. It was time to push! There was no time to reapply the oils; the ones that were applied before bedtime would have to suffice.

Having used my YL oils, I felt so relaxed that it only took three swift pushes and our baby girl, Faith Moriah Douglas, was born at 4:10 a.m., only one hour and 10 minutes after arriving at the hospital. Moments after her birth, Chris placed her on my chest, and we anointed her in the name of the Lord Jesus with the following oils diluted with equal parts of V-6™ oil:

• Brain Power™, which includes frankincense oil in it that stimulates the limbic part of the brain and helps to overcome stress, was put on Faith's head.
• Valor®, which also has frankincense oil, was placed on her spine.
• Joy™, which includes rose oil that contains the highest frequency among essential oils, was placed over her heart.
• Peace & Calming®, containing orange and ylang ylang oils and increases relaxation, was placed on her feet.
• Lavender, a great relaxant, was used as a whole body message.

I continued using the YL oils on myself and Faith and never suffered a bout of postpartum depression. I call this "my perfect home birth in a hospital." To this day, Faith still enjoys being rubbed with these stellar YL essential oils. To God be all the glory! God's richest blessings on you and your precious baby.

Beverly Boytim, mother to four
My two-year-old touched a hot generator muffler. We were a good way from our house and my husband put his hand under cold water while I ran to the house for lavender. When I got back my son was in hysterics. I applied the lavender to his hand, and he calmed down considerably. We then took him to the house and continued with cold water and lavender. When the burning sensation had finally abated, I sprayed his hand with LavaDerm™ and applied a homemade burn paste; I then wrapped the hand in an ace bandage. Everyday, I would let the burn get some air and then spray again and apply the paste. Three days later, the burn was healed and about 10 days later there was no sign of it.

I had a huge fear of pushing to the point that my midwife told me I held the birth of my third child about two hours just because I was afraid to push. I did not want this with my fourth, and I asked my naturopath what oils she thought would be good. I used Surrender™ and Release™ during the last three months, and I applied them to my wrist daily and smelled them. I did not have time to diffuse them during my labor though; it only lasted three hours with about five minutes of pushing.

Sera Johnson, mother to four
I am so blessed to have had my surprise oil baby, Ethan! This was my fourth pregnancy and was by far the best ever. Despite dealing with nausea the first trimester, — peppermint became my best friend — overall I felt better than ever. Because of the NingXia Red®, Core Supplements, essential oils and a healthy diet, my energy stayed up, I didn't have any swelling, and my weight gain was less than my other pregnancies. The biggest difference was feeling so great overall. All of my labors and deliveries were short, but this one was the shortest and easiest — under two hours and I only pushed a few times. The most interesting thing was that my midwife commented that my placenta was one of the healthiest she had ever seen. Also, the nurse assistant noted that I had very rich milk.

Ethan was born with a condition called Torticollis where the muscles on the left side of his neck were too short and tight due to him being so big and being stuck in a certain position in utero. His head tilted to the left, and he had a bit of a droopy left eye. We didn't think much of it until he was about four months old and he still wouldn't hold his head totally straight up. A midwife knew exactly what it was and recommended I take him to a pediatric wellness chiropractor. I had never heard of this before, so I researched and found that if not corrected, it could cause physical developmental delays. With treatment, I learned it would take six months to a year to correct. So we started using the essential oils, particularly Valor®, peppermint and PanAway® along with the chiropractic, and, in two months, his head was totally straight and the muscles where perfect! Praise the Lord!

I really feel like a better mom now. Whenever anyone asks me if essential oils are okay for newborns and infants, I say, "Absolutely!" To God be the Glory! We are so blessed!

Wendy Stanziano, mother to two
Young Living Essential Oils and products have made such a difference in our lives and in the kind of mother I am becoming. Unfortunately, I didn't know much about the oils until after I had our first child, but, since Caleb came home, we've used lavender to help him sleep. After successfully relieving Caleb's RSV at three months of age, the oils have been an amazing tool for all the mild ailments infants have. To this day, I use Thieves® and R.C.™ for our whole family at the slightest sign of a cold and lavender for any burns or skin irritation. My husband used the Thyromin™ for an underactive thyroid and has normal hormone levels today. I am currently using Thyromin™ and EndoFlex™ for my own hyperactive thyroid.

In addition to the oils, I believe that the NingXia Red® has been an integral part of our health and wellness by building my whole family's immune systems.

A few days before we were going out of town to see family, I noticed red bumps/blisters on my son's feet. Because Caleb had slept terribly the night before, I immediately suspected hand-foot-and-mouth disease. I checked his hands and mouth for blisters but couldn't find any. He didn't have a fever or other symptoms. I chalked it up to teething.

By lunchtime, he had developed the blisters on his hands. I still didn't see any in his mouth, but I knew it had to be the virus, especially when he wouldn't eat solids for dinner that night. I alternated with mountain savory and Purification®.

Just an hour or so after applying the Purification®, I tried to show the bumps to my mom, and I could only find two! I kept applying the Purification® at every diaper change on Monday. By Wednesday, the bumps were gone from his hands and only red spots remained on his feet! He never seemed to have the fever, but the Purification® really seemed to have shortened the duration of the virus!

Caleb, now three years old, takes Young Living's daily vitamin for children, KidScents® MightyVites, along with NingXia Red®. He's rarely at the doctor and avoided any type of antibiotic until this past winter. We also use the KidScents® bath products on him and on our newest addition, Ava Rose. In fact, at just a few weeks old, Ava showed signs of a cold and congestion, which responded well to a little R.C.™ and Thieves® in the diffuser. It's a great feeling to know that I have the power to use God's natural healing methods on my children! So many coughs, colds, tummy aches, and fevers have been alleviated with the various YL oils in the past three years.

Laura Hopkins, first-time mother
Young Living's therapeutic-grade essential oils are amazing because I can use them on my daughter, my husband, myself and even on our dog, without side effects. As I began to learn about them, I realized that God purposefully designed nature to provide these healing agents for us, His children. How loved and blessed we are! Unlike man's medicine, God created these oils to correct the root of a problem — infection, fungus, parasites — as well as the symptoms — fever, running nose, constipation.

My first experience was when my four-month-old, Audrey, developed a fever. I used peppermint diluted 50-50 with V-6™ oil in her belly button. Almost immediately, it helped her have a bowel movement and reduced her fever, so I continued the regime every three hours. I also put Valor® on her spine, and she was back to normal later that day.

Before eating, Audrey takes both her MightyZymes and her MightyVites three times a day. She also starts each day with at least one ounce of NingXia Red® and loves to put on orange, Purification® and Peace & Calming®. Between these products and oils and the Scriptures we confess about good health, she has never been to the doctor's office for anything other than a well-baby appointment. We have witnessed hundreds of testimonies in the past few years with family and friends of all ages. God is good all the time!

Jeanette Watje, mother to eight
I love to hear my two-year-old say, "Mommy oils, oils" and lie down with her feet up in the air! It also is hilarious seeing my teenagers crawl up the stairs, so they don't waste any oil on their socks and can go to sleep with oils on their feet. None of my eight children have been seriously sick in over two years! We go places and are not in fear of getting sick, but, if we do, we are well within days instead of weeks like others that have the same sickness. We are praising God that we are feeling better and finding not only quick fixes but also preventive maintenance, too. Instead of testimonies, I call these victories!

When someone is sick, it is a ritual for all my kids to line up with their socks off at night and lie down so I can oil their feet, backs and sometimes chests depending on their illness. It is a blessing to see my children, who catch on quicker than I do, go to the oils first to solve health issues that occur. It is amazing to see God provide healing of so many things with the oils.

Kim Spendlove, mother to five

My fourth child was delivered via C-section, leaving me with an inverted "T" C-section scar; the surgery left me severely anemic, and my recovery was very difficult. I did not know about YL essential oils at the time. After hearing the news we could never have another natural birth, my husband had a vasectomy. We immediately regretted it, and a year later the Lord made a reversal possible. We conceived our fifth child shortly after the reversal and once again were faced with the issue of our birthing options. Desperate to avoid another C-section, we wanted to do everything we could to heal the wound. A year and a half had gone by, but we decided to try cistus and lavender applied over the womb area nightly to see what it would do.

I delivered our baby, a beautiful little girl in May 2008. We had a perfect natural VBAC without any complication. In fact, it was the easiest one so far. Even though we have no way of seeing my internal scar, the fading of my external one is substantial, and the pain and sensitivity I had are completely resolved. While I know oils were not the only factor, I am confident they played a key role in helping my womb to regenerate and strengthen making our VBAC possible.

I was in labor for 27 hours, and, while it went very well, it was also extremely tiring. Several times when my energy was fading, we rubbed Valor® on my inner ankles. Within minutes I felt renewed and joyful, and any doubts that were trying to creep in faded away. As we neared transition, my husband applied peppermint to my spine. I had a total of three transition contractions. The last one sent me from nine centimeters to 10, broke my water and sent our baby girl on her way into the world. Within a couple minutes and two pushes, she was born. It was the fastest, easiest delivery I have ever had.

When my nursing newborn doesn't like something I have eaten, I apply Peace & Calming® over her tummy. Within about 10 minutes she relaxes and her spitting up stops completely. It usually doesn't return for the rest of the night.

Becky Madding, R.N. B.S.N., mother to four

I am a white female whose weight has always been within the acceptable range for my height. I eat fairly healthy (never eat fried foods, rarely fast food, minimal sweets), I am active (keeping up with three toddlers and walking ¾ mile every night). No one in my family has ever had Type 1 diabetes, no one has ever had gestational diabetes, but I do have two aunts that have recently been diagnosed with Type 2 diabetes, and both are on medications for it. With my pregnancies I have never gained more than 20 pounds and typically it was less than 15 pounds. Basically, I had zero risk factors for becoming a gestational diabetic.

When I failed my first glucose tolerance test with my first child, my doctor was stunned. My numbers were high but not so bad that medications or insulin were ever considered. I controlled my diet easily, and my glucose ranged usually from 80 to the 120s. Occasionally, I would be high, but my glucose never went above 130s.

I managed to not have gestational diabetes with my second and third children. However, with my fourth, I failed the tolerance test terribly. By this time, the only risk factor beside my previous diagnosis was my age; I was 35 years old with the fourth versus 30 with my first. I failed so badly that my doctor wanted to put me on insulin immediately. The diabetic educators talked him into giving me a two-week, diet-controlled trial before going that route. When I initially started on the diet, I was finding it impossible to keep my numbers down. This time my highs were in the 180s, and

I was out of range at least once a day but more often twice a day. I was so frustrated and had to almost starve myself to keep my sugars down, as best I could. I was absolutely fearful that I would have to go on insulin.

Then, I got my NingXia Red®. I started taking one ounce three times a day, following each meal. Within three to four days, I noticed a dramatic difference. My sugars were in range (less than 120) almost all the time. I was usually high once or twice a week after starting NingXia Red®, but, when I was high, it was only in the 130s not the 180s. After a week, I noticed that I was able to eat larger portions and still maintain my sugars within range. That is awesome when you are pregnant and hungry almost all the time! I could not have done it without NingXia Red®. Being diabetic while pregnant carries with it a lot of added risks both for mother and child, but, if it can be diet controlled and controlled well, the risks decrease markedly. I had a healthy, eight pound baby girl, full term with zero complications. Praise God!

Christa Smith, mother to 14
My first nine deliveries were induced due to preeclampsia or pregnancy-induced hypertension (PIH). The doctors used medications to control my high blood pressure, but usually it quit working at 32 weeks. I tried several medications, but I had to be induced because my body was so toxic — high ketones in my urine and high blood pressure that measured as high as 190/160. I spent most of my pregnancies on bed rest and was hospitalized at 31 weeks and given magnesium sulfate to keep my muscles from contracting and prevent pre-term labor. I had such horrible migraines, just sitting up would cause my blood pressure to rise. Typically, I was on the medications two months before and two months after delivering.

Early in my eleventh pregnancy, I attended an essential oils class. I was interested in what the oils could do for my two-year-old who struggled with allergies that caused severe breathing problems. It was so severe that my daughter was on all fours coughing and trying to catch her breath. I made a rectal implant/enema with oils recommended for bronchitis. I watched her get up and start playing within 10 seconds. To God be the glory!

About 38 weeks along in my eleventh pregnancy, my midwife found I again had high ketones in my urine and learned I was hypoglycemic. Facing another induction and possible C-section, I began a protocol of ingesting coriander, dill, peppermint, lavender and fennel oils and a nutrition plan with Power Meal, JuvaPower®, Life 5™ Probiotic, Omega Blue™ (now known as OmegaGize3™) and Pure Protein Complete™. I was shocked one week later with the results. Not only did the oils help, but I had no ketones in my urine and was no longer toxic.

My eleventh delivery was an amazing, natural, vaginal birth. I used the oils recommended in *Gentle Babies* throughout labor, and we anointed our son with frankincense as soon as he was born. I also put myrrh on his umbilical cord, and it fell off within 24 hours.

Our home hasn't been the same since we began using God's oils. I diffuse cedarwood for congestion and sinus issues. We've gotten rid of warts with frankincense, relieved congestion with Thieves®, peppermint and cedarwood, and dealt with sores with lavender and balsam fir. When you have 14 children, you can really test the oils. I know Young Living has the best products because there is nothing at our house that they can't handle.

Evon McDonald, mother to 3 and grandmother to 8
Our grandson Noah was given to us by the courts at the age of three months. Between two and three years of age, it was hard to watch our new son begin

to exhibit signs of autism. Our first clues were what we thought was a lack of bonding with us. He did not want to be held, wanted to be alone and would not look at people when they tried to talk with him. As he neared three years of age, he became obsessive. The only way to get his attention was to touch him. He appeared to live in his own little world. He saw his regular doctor very, very often for sore throats, congestion, runny noses and earaches and seemed to be on antibiotics every few weeks. Our doctor saw the possibility of autism in his behavior and sent him to a specialist, who confirmed our fears after evaluating him.

A friend suggested I research essential oils instead of all the antibiotics he was taking. After research, we realized that Young Living products were the best available. We began by putting two drops of Thieves® on his feet every night; we used R.C.™ on his chest for congestion and peppermint in his navel for a temperature.

We put frankincense above his eyebrows and Brain Power™ on his temples every morning before he left for school. Between ages four and five, he only saw his doctor a handful of times.

Noah is very intelligent. He memorizes anything he hears and can repeat extensive dialogues of movies. By the age of four, he could count to 150 by 2s, 5s and 10s, knew his phonic sounds and could spell over 40 words including all of the colors. However he would not hold a pencil to learn to write. He would talk to himself for hours while playing, but his vocabulary was memorized movie dialogues. He could not tell us if he was hungry or thirsty and was not potty trained at age five. He did not react to pain nor could he tell us where he hurt, but he angered easily.

In January 2009, I read about children with starving brains and learned how gluten binds to the receptors in the intestines and starves the brain by preventing the nutrients from being absorbed. After researching and going to the YL Convention, I realized YL had developed a product called MightyZymes that supplies a child's body with enzymes to breakdown many things, including gluten. I started giving Noah MightyZymes, but it was a hit and miss proposition. We did see improvement. He became more loving, wanted to be held and began to come and get us by the hand and take us somewhere to get something for him. In April 2009, he no longer wore a diaper during the day. He had very few accidents even at school and began to ask people their names.

In May 2009, I committed to give him three MightyZymes each day, every day. By the end of June, he burst out of his shell. His first sentence just blew me away: "Mommy, cook me some food." I knew that was not from a movie. He began talking in a conversational method and wanted us with him, to play, watch movies and read with him. During the first part of July, we quit putting a night diaper on him. In January 2010, we had multiple family emergencies that disrupted our daily routine of applying oils and giving Noah MightyZymes. We began to notice regression in several areas and so did his teachers. This reinforced my belief that through YL's MightyZymes and essential oils, our Heavenly Father had released our child from many of the daily struggles of autism. I am recommitted to our previous habits of using YL products and am so blessed that we are all His children! (Matthew 6:33)

About the Author

Debra Raybern shares her passion for health and wellness in the healing and restoring power of God's medicine, natural herbs, essential oils, right relationships and nutrition through seminars, lectures, books and magazine articles. Her vast knowledge, experience and Godly anointing has allowed her the privilege to help countless people with both minor and life threatening health problems by educating them in healthy nutrition practices, lifestyle, herbs and essential oils to cleanse and promote the body to heal itself.

Debra is certified in various holistic modalities, including naturopathy through the Herbal Healer Academy, a Master Herbalist Degree from The School of Natural Healing, as a Internationally Certified Aromatherapist by the Pacific Institute of Aromatherapy and as a Certified Nutritional Counselor with the American Association of Nutritional Counselors. She writes, lectures and teaches on the safe and effective use of herbs, herbal preparation methods and therapeutic-grade essential oils, as well as a variety of natural health topics. Debra's wellness articles have appeared in publications such as *Countryside*, *Home School Digest*, *The Old Schoolhouse*, *The Link* and *An Encouraging Word*. Her video, *Whole Grain Cooking*, and the recipe collection, *From Our House To Your House*, have helped many in preparing nutritious and delicious healthy meals. In 2009, she co-authored the ground-breaking book that serves as a family health program and curriculum *Nutrition 101: Choose Life!*

Gentle Babies Reference and Resource List

Along with the hundreds of testimonies for happy moms using essential oils, these are just a few of the many books and resources I have learned from that have been used to write this book:

100 Herb Syllabus, Dr. John R. Christopher, Christopher Publications, 1996

The ABC Clinical Guide to Herbs, Mark Blumenthal, The American Botanical Council, 2003

Advanced Aromatherapy, Kurt Schnaubelt, PhD, 1995, Healing Arts Press, Rochester, Vermont

Aromatherapy Course, Part 1, Essential Oils, Kurt Schnaubelt, PhD, 1997

Aromatherapy for Health Professionals, Shirley & Len Price, Third Edition, 2007

A-Z Aromatherapy, Patricia Davis, 1998, Barnes & Noble Press

The Chemistry of Essential Oils Made Simple, David Stewart, Ph. D., D.N.M., Care Publications, 2005

Clinical Aromatherapy, Jane Buckle, RN, Ph. D, Second Edition, Churchill Livingstone

Essential Oils Desk Reference Guide, Editions 2,3,4,and 5, Life Science Publishing

Healing Oils Healing Hands, Linda L. Smith, RN, MS, HNC, HTCP, CHHP, CCA, HTSM Press, 2008

The Healing Intelligence of Essential Oils, Kurt Schnaubelt, PhD, 2011

Healing Oils of the Bible, David Stewart, Ph. D., D.N.M., Care Publications, 2005

Herbs of the Bible, James A. Duke, Ph. D., Interweave Press, 1999

Medical Aromatherapy, Kurt Schnaubelt, PhD, 1999, North Atlantic Books

Moving Aromatherapy Forward, Kurt Schnaubelt, PhD, PIA Masters Series, 2004

Nature's Mold Rx, Edward R Close, Ph. D., Jacquelyn Close, RA, EJC Publications, 2007

Reference Guide for Essential Oils, Editions 9-12,Connie and Alan Higley, AbundantHealth4u.com

Releasing Emotional Patterns with Essential Oils, Carolyn L. Mein, DC, 1998

The School of Natural Healing, Dr. John R. Christopher, 1996, Christopher Publications

Plus over 250 books and more than 500 hours of video and audio from:
The School of Natural Healing's Master Herbalist course, The Pacific Institute of Aromatherapy basic and masters courses, The Herbal Healer Academy's Herbal and Naturopath course and many other certification classes and seminars.

Resource Guide

Nutrition 101: Choose Life!

Growing Healthy Homes LLC offers this ground-breaking, family-friendly, Biblically-based curriculum co-authored by Debra Raybern. All ages can learn from this three-in-one family nutrition and health program that presents the major body systems, how they function, their common health issues, the benefits of good food and the consequences of bad food. Packed with hands-on activities, science and art projects and nearly 80 family-friendly recipes, this program teaches and reinforces the why's of what we should eat. The 448-page book also includes a complete reference guide filled with nutrition facts, charts, practical tips and an exhaustive index and serves as a constant resource for improved health and abundant living. Available in a CD-ROM, book or combo package. Review an excerpt and order online at www.GrowingHealthyHomes.com.

Essential Oils Desk Reference

The must have book for serious users of therapeutic-grade essential oils. It comes in two formats; large 500 page book or pocket size edition. The publisher, Life Science Publishing, also carries a large selection of other natural health books, brochures and other resources. To order online, visit www. lifesciencepublishing.com or call 1-800-336-6308 to request a catalog and order by phone.

Abundant Health 4 U

Abundant Health 4 U offers additional resources, accessories, oil bottles, droppers and oil carrying cases. To order online, visit www.abundanthealth4u.com.

ORDER YOUNG LIVING PRODUCTS

1. Make a list of the products you would like to purchase.
2. Have a credit card or debit card or check handy.
3. Call Young Living at 1-800-371-3515 or go online to www.youngliving.com to place your order. You must have an Enroller and/or Sponsor number. This is the person who shared this book with you or who first introduced you to Young Living Essential Oils.

- For online orders, first select your country, and then click on Sign Up. Follow the screen prompts by entering your personal information and the enroller/sponsor number.
- You may choose to become a general customer and pay retail or become an independent distributor buying at wholesale and saving 24 percent. There are no monthly obligations for purchasing or recruiting and no yearly membership renewal as an independent distributor; this can simply be a wholesale account for your personal purchases. If you desire, you may initiate a home-based business, but it is never required.
- If you select the customer option, make your purchases, and when the products arrive, enjoy!
- If you select Independent Distributor, select your kit. (The author suggests the Everyday Oils Kit, as it contains many of the oils mentioned in this book.) Then, select Continue Shopping to order other products or complete the ordering process.

4. Be sure to write down your new Young Living account number, personal identification number and password for future order. Then, wait for your products to arrive and enjoy!

To obtain additional copies of *Gentle Babies* and
for more information on other books by Growing
Healthy Homes, please visit our website at
www.GrowingHealthyHomes.com

Nutrition 101: Choose Life!

Gentle Babies Quick Reference Handout Pack

Gentle Babies DVD

The ABC's of Building a Young Living Organization

Young Living Skincare Product Handout Pack

Notes

Notes

Notes